cacao
addict

JOHN CROFT

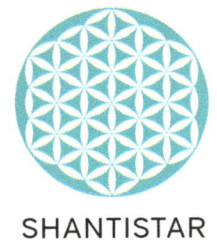

SHANTISTAR

AUTHOR
John Croft

RIGHT HAND MAN
Noel Blanchard

PHOTOGRAPHY & DESIGN
Natarsha Rawlins

COPY EDITOR
Emma Wheater

CONTACT
website www.shantistar.com
facebook www.facebook.com/shantistar
instagram shantistarcom
email om@shantistar.com

First Published in Western Australia
in 2018 by Vivid Publishing

All rights reserved. No part of this publication may be reproduced, stored in a retrieval system or transmitted in any form or by any means, electronic, mechanical, photocopying, recording or otherwise, without the prior written permission of the copyright holder.

Text Copyright © 2018 John Croft
Photography © 2018 Natarsha Rawlins

ISBN: 978-0-6457510-8-6

Printed on Demand in Australia,
UK and USA

Published by Vivid Publishing
A division of Fontaine Publishing Group
P.O. Box 948, Fremantle
Western Australia 6959
www.vividpublishing.com.au

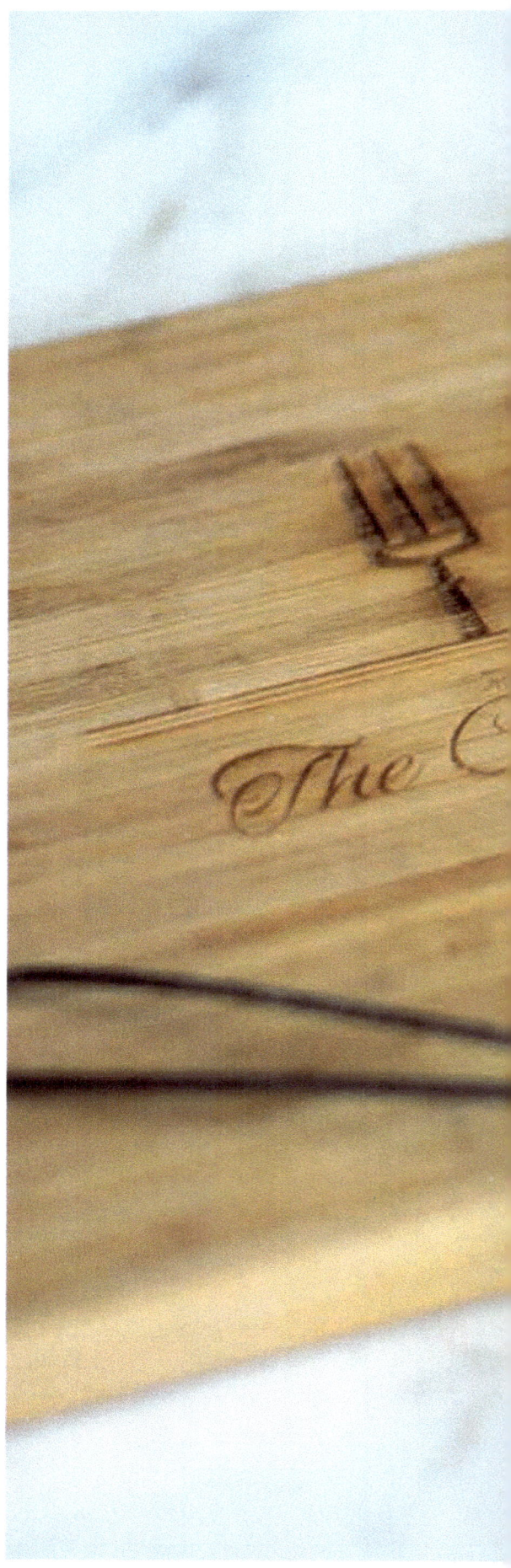

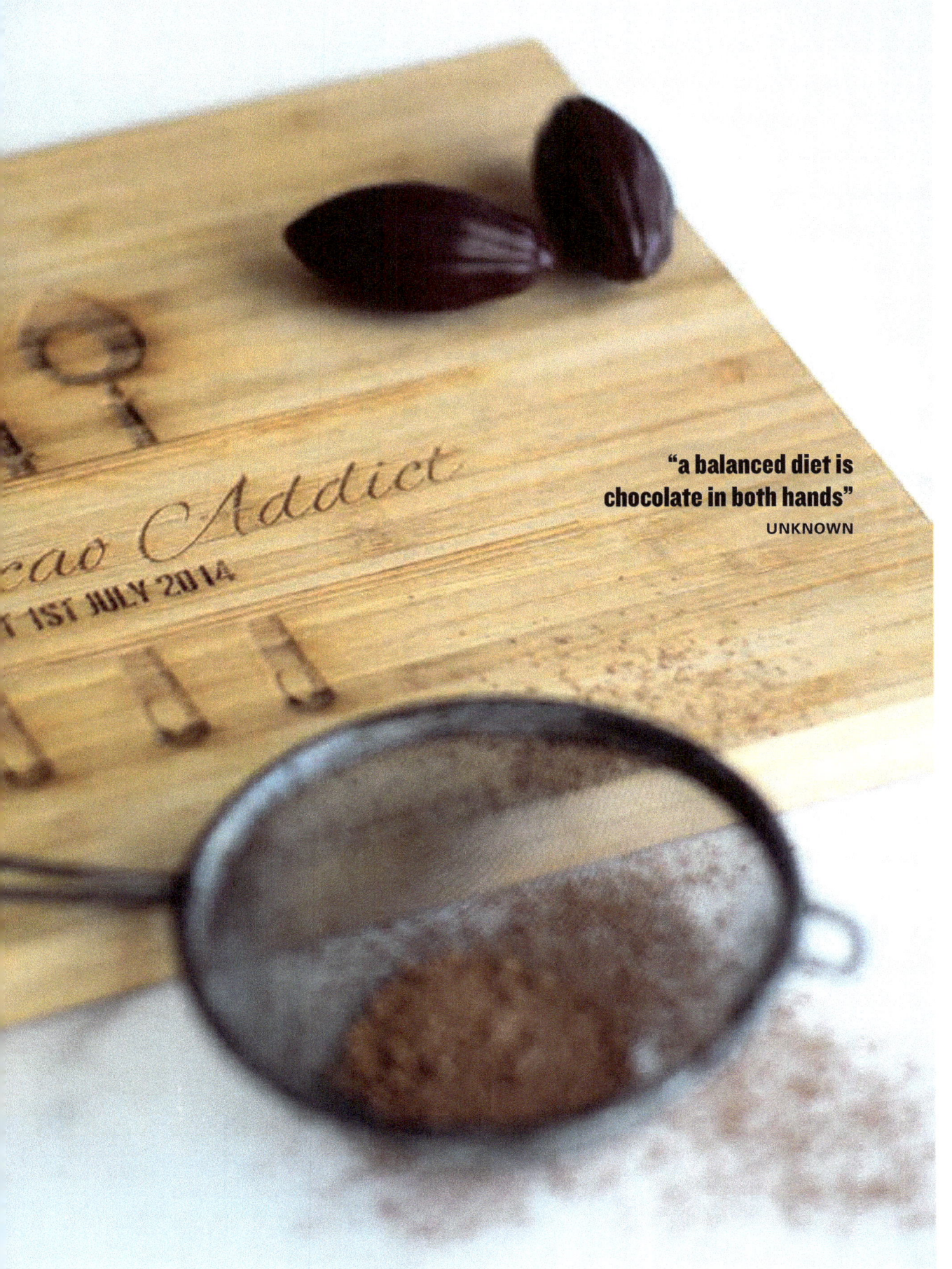

"a balanced diet is chocolate in both hands"
UNKNOWN

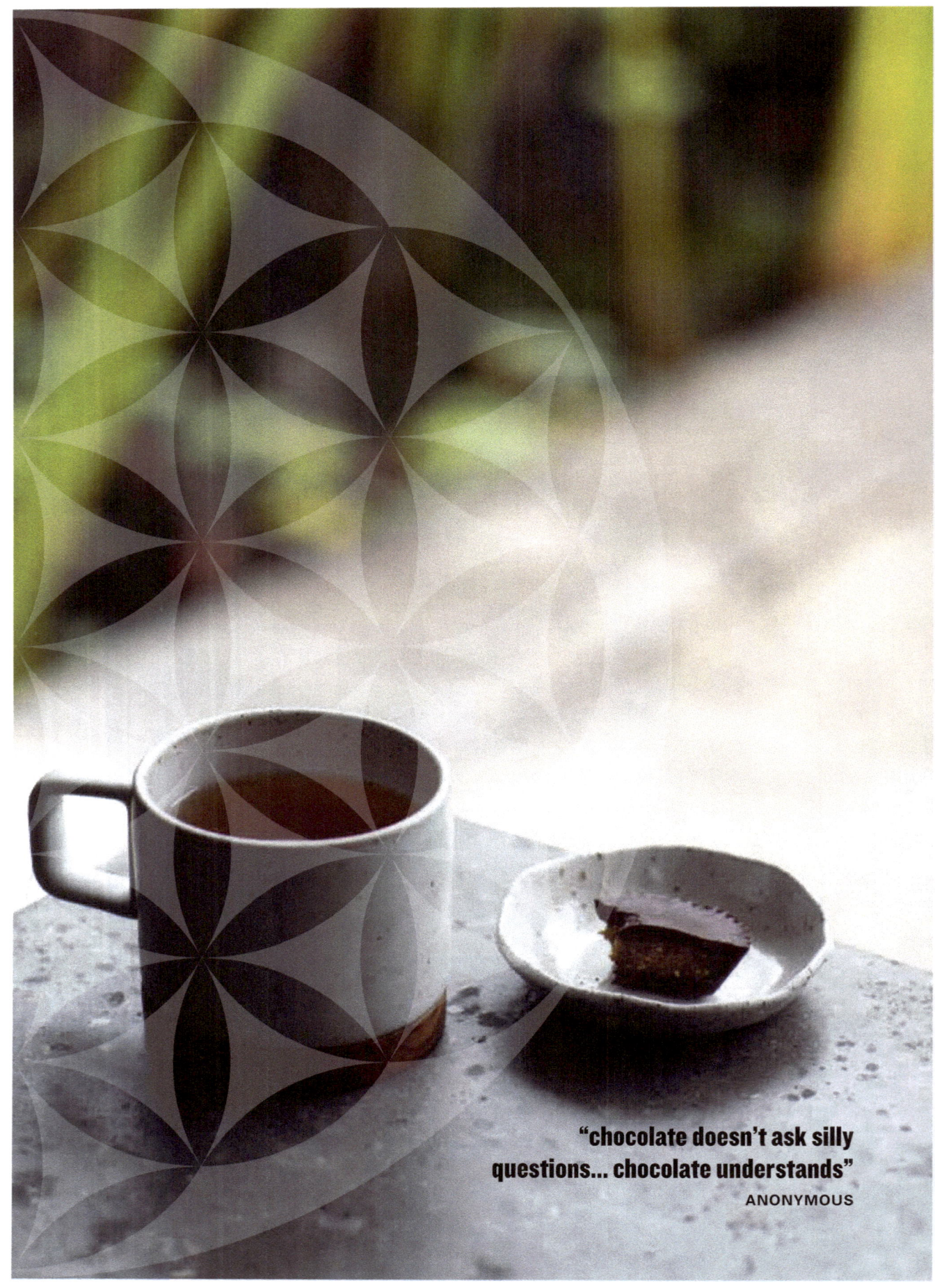

"chocolate doesn't ask silly questions... chocolate understands"
ANONYMOUS

WELCOME

I believe that food is medicine, and the healing power of food interests me immensely. Once revered as a currency in Mayan times, cacao offers a multitude of potent health benefits, which is why it is the star ingredient throughout **Cacao Addict**.

Tasting the "real deal" cacao many years ago (with many thanks to my cacao sister Vanessa Jean), opened my eyes up to what chocolate should taste like without all the sugar, dairy, low quality fats and processing that some commercial chocolate employs. Chocolate is supposed to make you feel good, but unfortunately a lot of commercial chocolate out there is far removed from what the ancients knew. Keep it simple, keep it real, and make it with good intentions.

Food should be adventurous, tantalizing and enjoyable, not only to the eye but especially the palette. My love of exotic places and travel has opened me up to wonderful spices, smells, tastes and ingredients from faraway places.

Superfoods from South America feature as additions in many of my recipes. Ingredients such as acai, lucuma, camu camu, maca, medicinal mushroom powder, vanilla and maqui not only add interest, but so many health-giving properties too. So, while these recipes look like decadent treats, you're not eating something empty and bad for you, but rather something that is nourishing, satisfying and whole. The addition of so many superfoods and (food grade) essential oils takes these cacao creations to medicinal heights.

Myself and my partner Noel have been immersed in the natural health world for over 30 years and in our cooking classes it is very much a shared experience – I might be the one at the front who is getting their hands messy, but everyone in the room contributes to the end product through their energy, interest and presence. We cook, meditate and eat together, but in reality, it is more than this. The experience goes beyond simply making something to eat. It is nurturing, healing, and creates community. To extend the physical community that has been created in our home in Western Australia, I invite you to help us create a larger community that reaches around the world by tagging us with your creations – whether that is a recipe from this book, or one of your own invention. Find us @shantistarcom and use #cacaoaddict so we can share in your cacao journey.

With love,
John (& Noel)

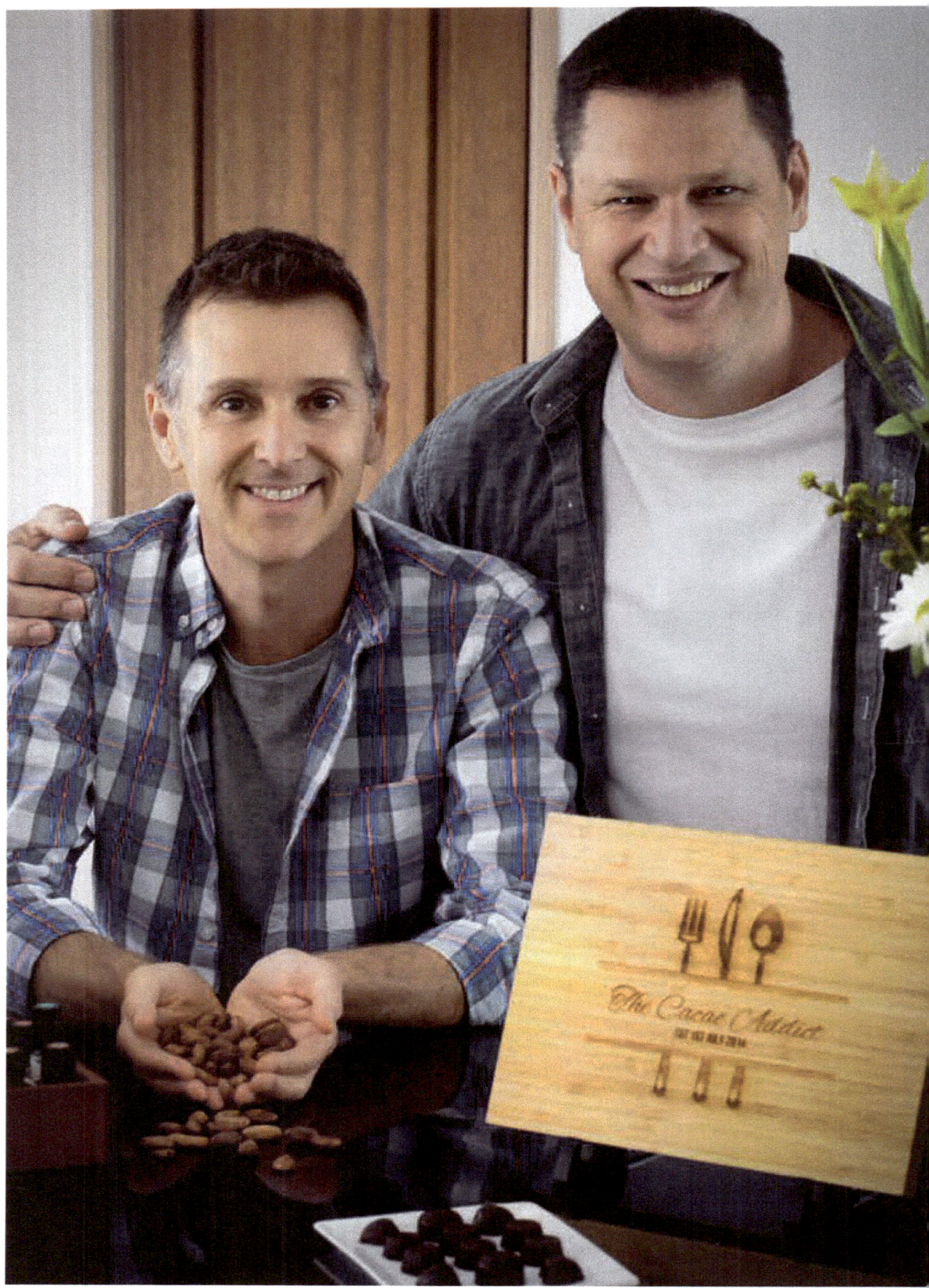

JUST THE TWO OF US

I grew up in Western Australia, in an Italian/Australian family. My love for good food was instilled by my mother, who always prepared the most fresh and amazing meals for us – and still does. For me, Hippocrates' quote "let food be thy medicine and medicine be thy food" really says it all (I think he was talking about chocolate!).

When I left school I wanted to travel the world, meet great people in exotic places and go on adventures, and by then my desire for eating good food with style and flavour was just second nature. I was interested in the healing arts, and decided to pursue a career in disability work.

Looking back, it all makes sense where we have ended up now.

Noel grew up in rural areas of Western Australia and travelled the state extensively with his family. He completed a chef apprenticeship, and in what now feels like a previous life, he was also a commercial real estate agent before training in hypnotherapy and NLP.

We met in 1994, and began a discovery of meditation, world travel, mindfulness, music, healing, sound therapy and raw chocolate. Yummm, right?

Our focus is aligned with helping people to connect with their own wellness journey through a healthy gut, mind and body. For us this also includes nourishing the mind and spirit through travel and eating great food from all over the world, as well as including pure essential oils into our daily routine to support our body and emotions. Pure essential oils are very powerful facilitators of change, and we have experienced this firsthand.

We've always been interested in spirituality and how living a natural well-balanced and healthy lifestyle, can help align the mind, body and spirit. We facilitate regular meditations, raw chocolate classes, and deliver a massage technique utilising dōTERRA's essential oils, called Aromatouch.

So together we strive to create a community of togetherness, wellness, inspiration, and have an holistic approach to living a balanced life. Our bigger vision is to educate and empower people to learn about options, choices and a better way of living, that involves a network of connection, great chocolate, pure essential oils, sound and helping to change mindset, on what we ALL can achieve in this life.

We continue in gratitude to travel and facilitate workshops on all areas of an holistic approach to health – whilst still enjoying wine and espresso martinis in moderation – we hope to inspire others to do the same and enjoy their abundant life.

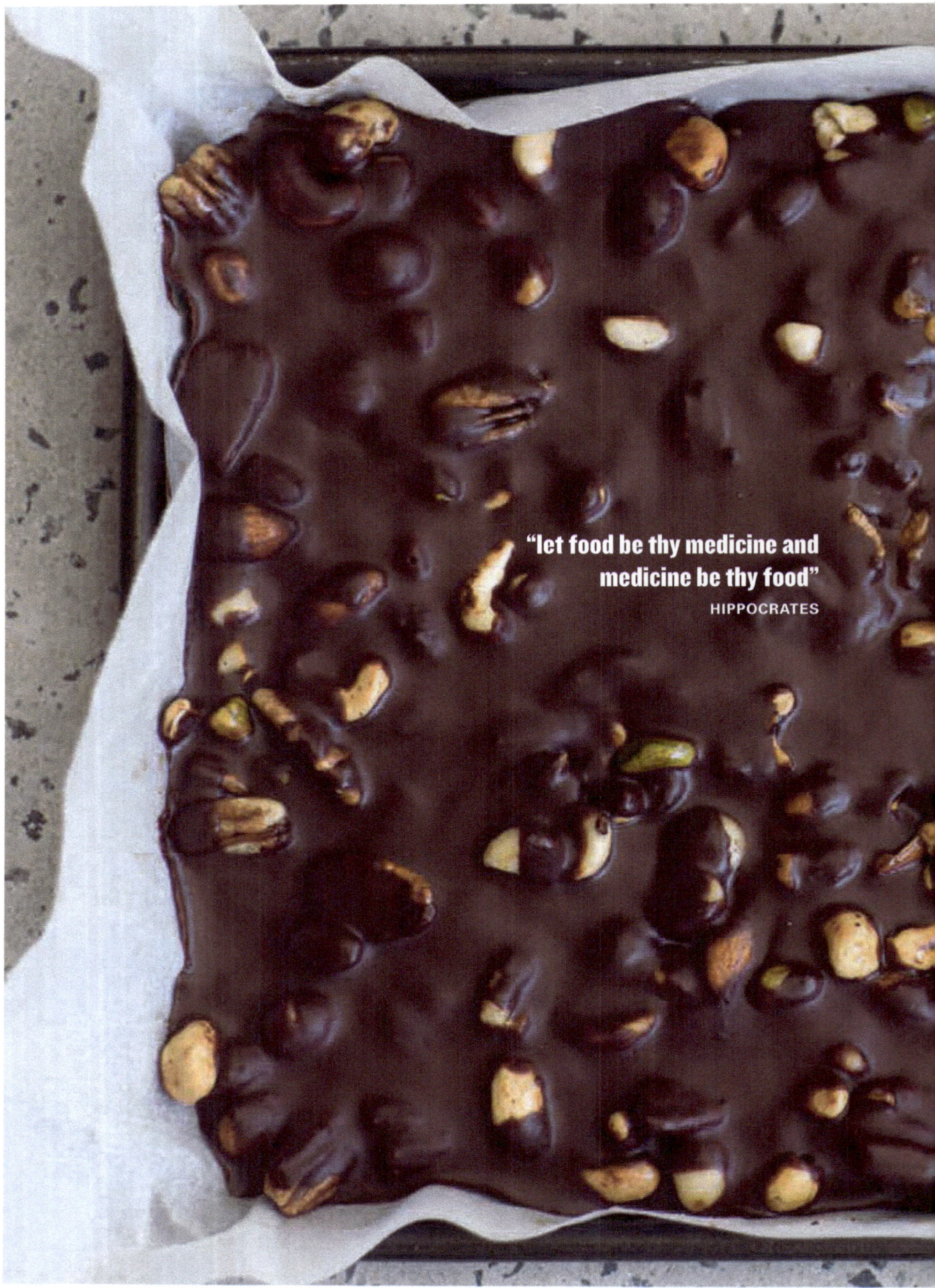

> "let food be thy medicine and medicine be thy food"
>
> HIPPOCRATES

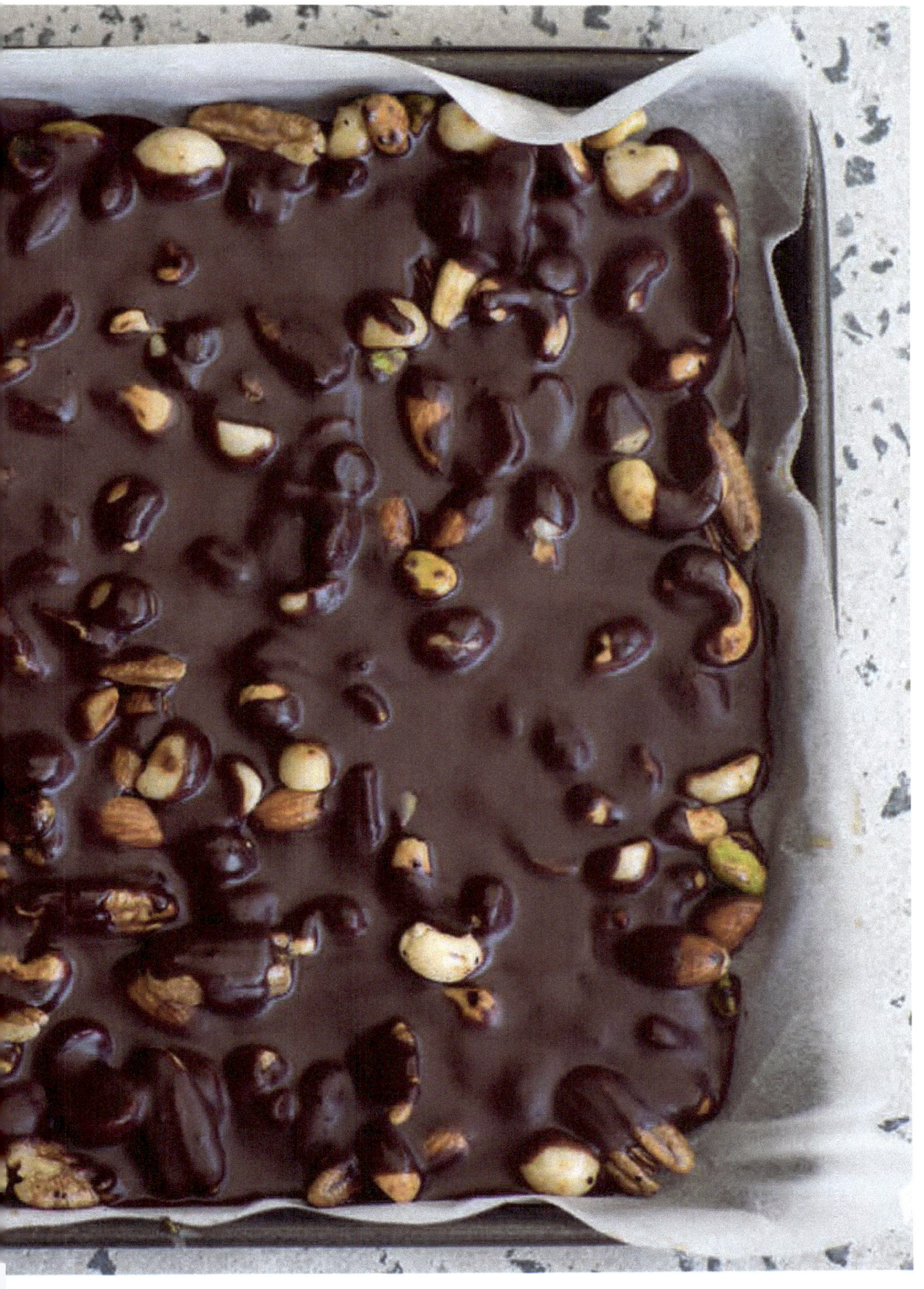

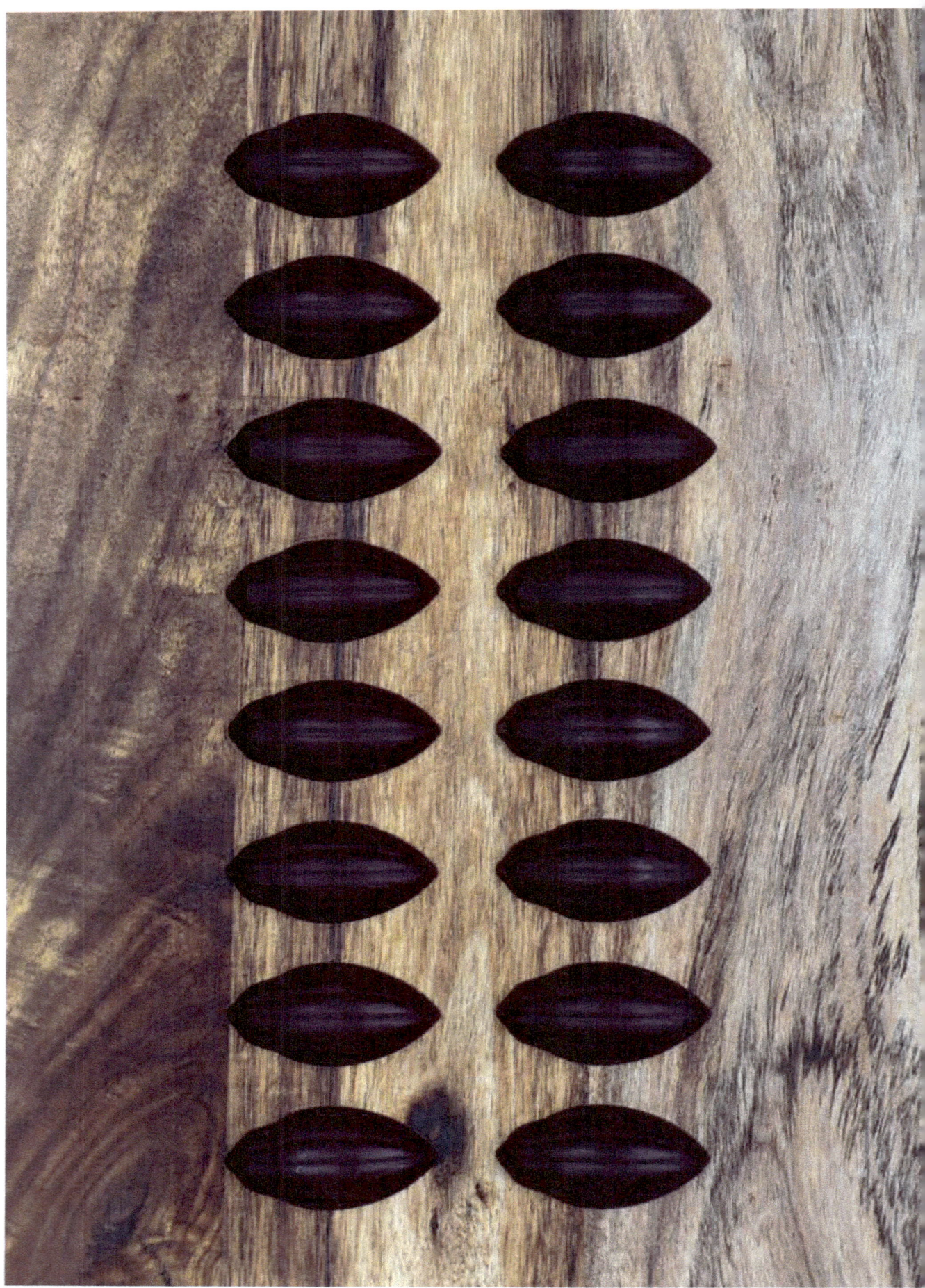

CACAO

I love the versatility of cacao. It can be used in sweet and savoury dishes, and comes in many different forms. It's a staple for many cultures around the world and is loved, craved for and even worshipped by many. In Mayan times it was valued as a form of currency, and was used in ceremonies – in pure, high doses it delivers a euphoric effect, as well as heightened awareness and connectedness. The name Theobroma Cacao literally translates to "food of the gods".

I have been lucky to travel to many places that grow cacao (but not Peru – yet!) and have witnessed their cacao plantations and trees. They are quite a surreal plant: the colours of the pods range from yellows to greens, to reds and oranges and look quite exotic and unusual.

The importance of sourcing good quality cacao for me personally is so essential, as some countries do not do this ethically, sustainably and often children are used as cheap labour with very unfair working conditions. I always choose an organic, ethically-sourced Peruvian cacao.

There are many, many different cacao cultivars out there, but in my experience and opinion, South America, namely Peru, grows the best cacao. Peru's climate, soil and altitude are so well suited to growing cacao, it really does make a difference to the chemistry and taste. Cacao releases chemicals in the brain like anandamide, serotonin and dopamine, which in turn give you the chocolate buzz feeling. It is also high in magnesium, antioxidants, vitamins, minerals, calcium and iron. So when combined with superfood powders and food-grade essential oils, it's a powerhouse snack loaded with many nutrients and health benefits.

These recipes can be enjoyed simply as a delicious experience, or you can delve deep into researching the various ingredients and discover the incredible healing properties that these foods contain. When you can, choose the best possible grade of ingredient available to you. Healing comes not just from the ingredients, but how they are treated and combined, and what energy you put into the food when you make it.

Essential oils throughout this book

Most, if not all, of these recipes use essential oils. This is because they bring a depth of flavour that elevates the taste and experience of making and consuming these treats to a totally different level, and they offer myriad health benefits. We use essential oils throughout our home for many and varied applications, so it made perfect sense to extend their pure qualities to the cacao treats I create.

Essential oils, like many products, vary greatly in their quality. I choose dōTERRA pure essential oils exclusively because I know they are of the highest grade available. If you want to use them too, go to our website shantistar.com where you can find more information. Not all oils are designed to be taken internally, so make sure that whatever you use is food-grade.

We have been using essential oils collectively for over 30 years but were honestly so amazed by the notable difference of dōTERRA's oils in terms of purity and grade. We had only really been using them for the scent and for meditation space in the past, but since being introduced to dōTERRA's oils nearly 4 years ago, they have become a big part of our lives for emotional, spiritual and physical health in so many ways.

The real difference with what we had been using previously and now, is that dōTERRA source their plant material from all around the world and where that plant grows best, working directly with the growers, and giving back so very much to their communities through sustainability practice, providing jobs, stability and financial remuneration. So at their core they are a company that not only makes the best oils on the planet, they care deeply about service, integrity, and giving back to communities all over the world. The testing that goes into every batch ensures the safety and purity that we had personally never seen with other oils that we had used in the past. The strength of dōTERRA's essential oils reflects in the amount needed for these recipes, less is best.

Quality oils can be an investment, so if you are starting a collection, choose a couple to start with, then enjoy the occasional treat of adding a new oil to your tool kit and expanding the treats you make and the experiences you can have with that oil in a diffuser at home, through massage, bathing, and so many more overall body system health applications. Like anything, you get what you pay for in terms of quality and purity, so don't opt for the cheapest you find. Do your research on the producer and get the best you can so you are giving yourself the best experience possible.

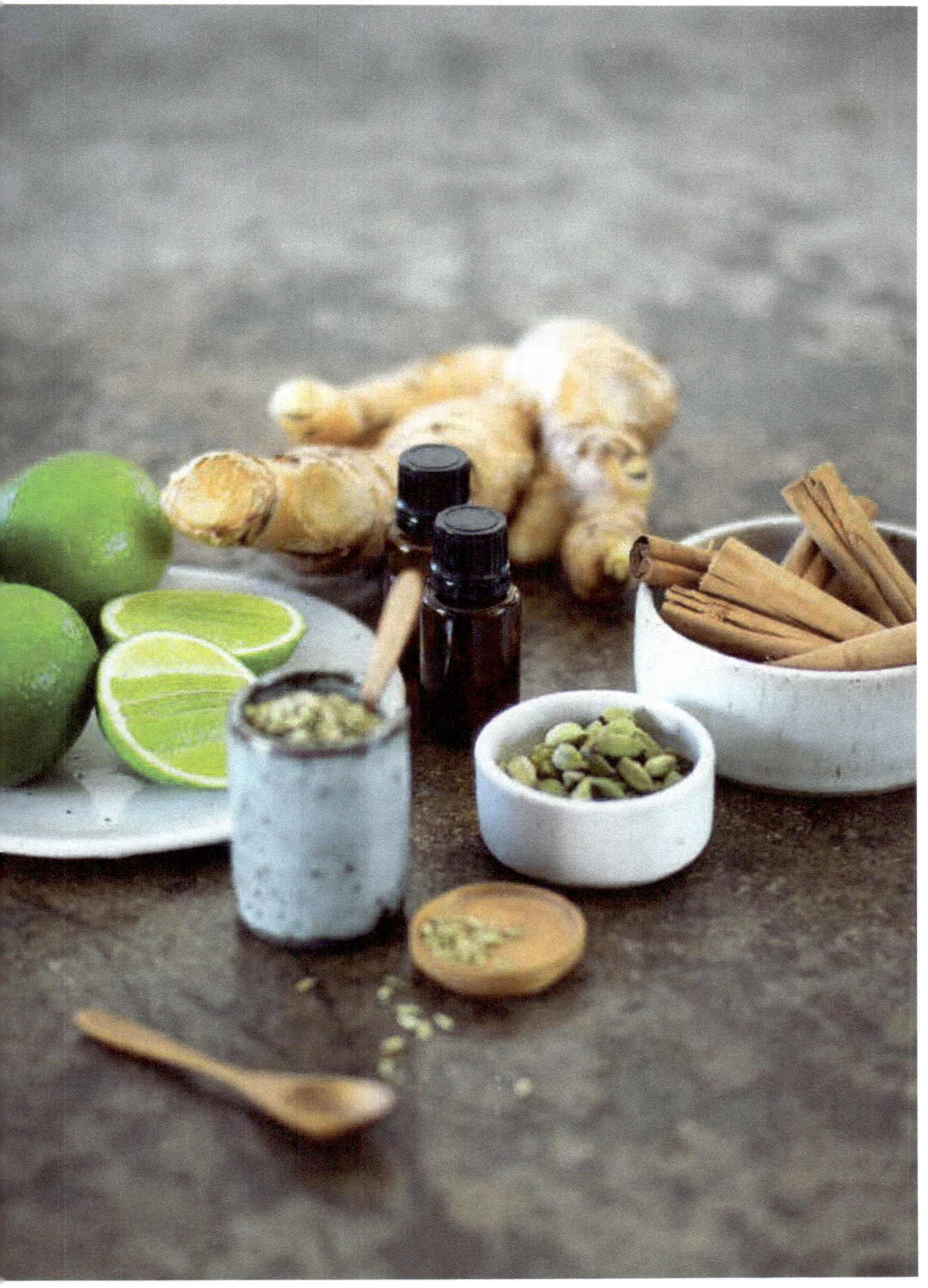

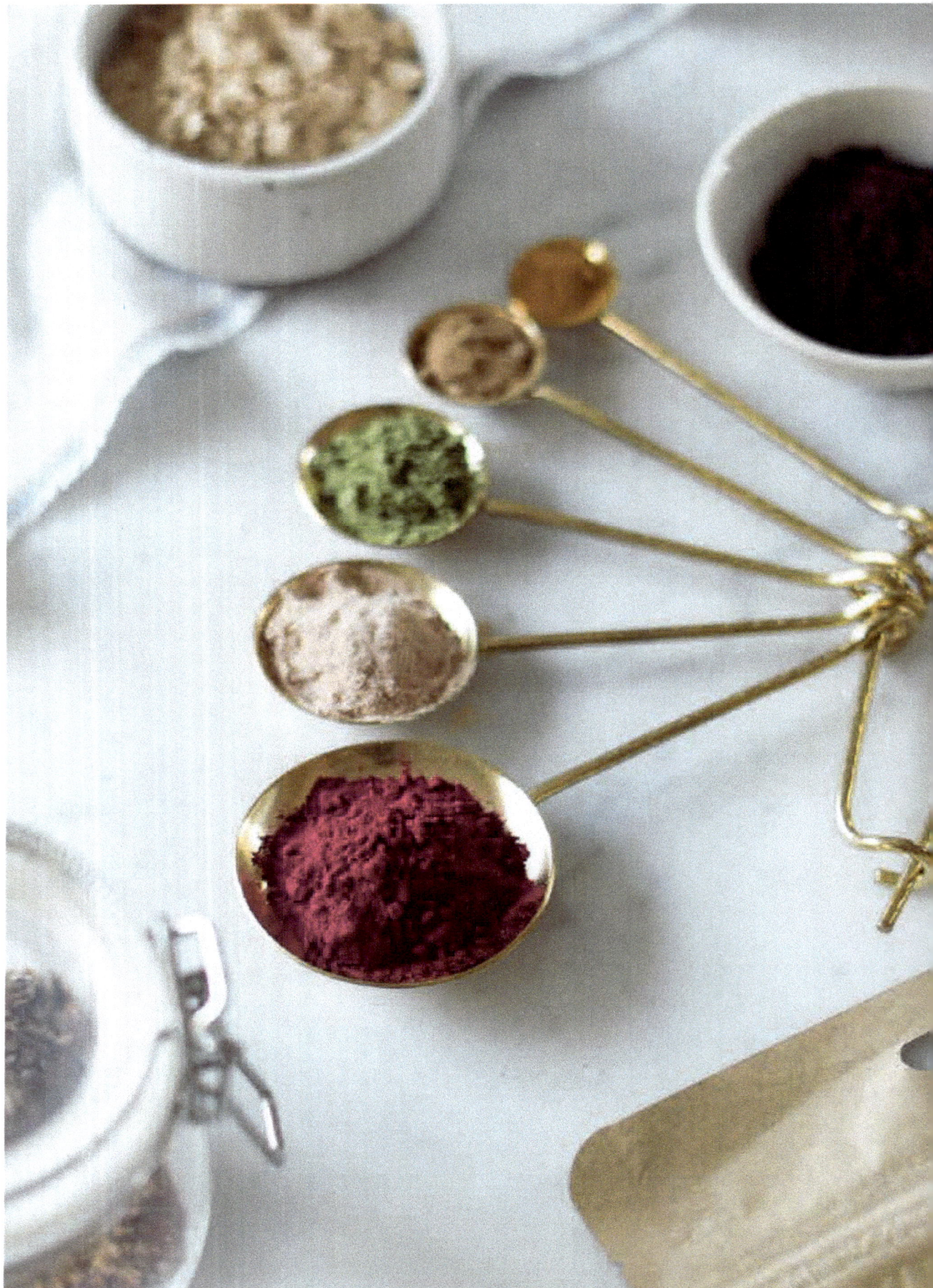

SUPERFOOD, SUPER GOOD

When I started making cacao creations, I wanted to create a synergy of raw cacao, superfood powders (mainly from South America) and food-grade essential oils, so with research, experimenting and sourcing good quality powders, I built up a collection that I add to different recipes, all for their different qualities and benefits. Many of these can be easily added to smoothies, slices and chocolate so experiment and see what you like best.

Superfood powders such as maca, lucuma, camu camu, maqui, acai and others can oxidise quickly, so I always leave them in the fridge to keep them fresh for longer.

TURMERIC A phenomenal anti-inflammatory anti-oxidant that is related to the ginger family that has been used in the Ayurvedic tradition for thousands of years. Turmeric generally needs fat and black pepper to make the curcumin more available to the body to absorb.

MACA This is probably one of my most used superfood powders, it has an almost malty flavour and is delicious in smoothies, biscuits and chocolate of course. It is known for supporting hormonal health, estrogen levels and male fertility.

LUCUMA Another exotic fruit out of Peru, it is a great source of fibre, and has many vitamins, minerals, and healthy carbohydrates.

CAMU CAMU Coming from another wonderful South American plant, the fruit from this plant produces such potent Vitamin C content, essential amino acids and anti-oxidative properties too.

MATCHA A beautiful, incredibly fine, green powder that comes from green tea leaves. Super high in antioxidant properties, essential polyphenols and a good dose of chlorophyll.

HEMP PROTEIN I love that hemp foods and products are becoming more readily available now and people are returning to this as a viable energy food source. Hemp protein is an amazing protein source for vegetarians and has good iron, magnesium and omegas essential for good body and brain health.

MAQUI A bright purple berry native to Chile, that is full of anti-ageing, anti-inflammatory and anti-oxidant benefits. I use it in powder form and add it to a lot of my recipes.

SPIRULINA A blue-green algae that has long been used as a protein, iron, and micronutrient source and is just full of amazing properties, such as detoxing heavy metals from your body, giving you an abundance of energy and assists in healthy cholesterol levels.

ACAI A deep purple berry from the Amazon that is a common addition to muesli and yoghurt bowls all over the world. It's a potent antioxidant and is full of vitamins and minerals, boosts mental function and like most berries, promotes a healthy metabolism.

MEDICINAL MUSHROOMS Long known for their "whole body system" health benefits throughout Asia for centuries, I love to play alchemist with these powders, cacao and essential oils making recipes for good health and vitality. I use a blend of many different varieties, working to boost immune, brain, heart, and organ health.

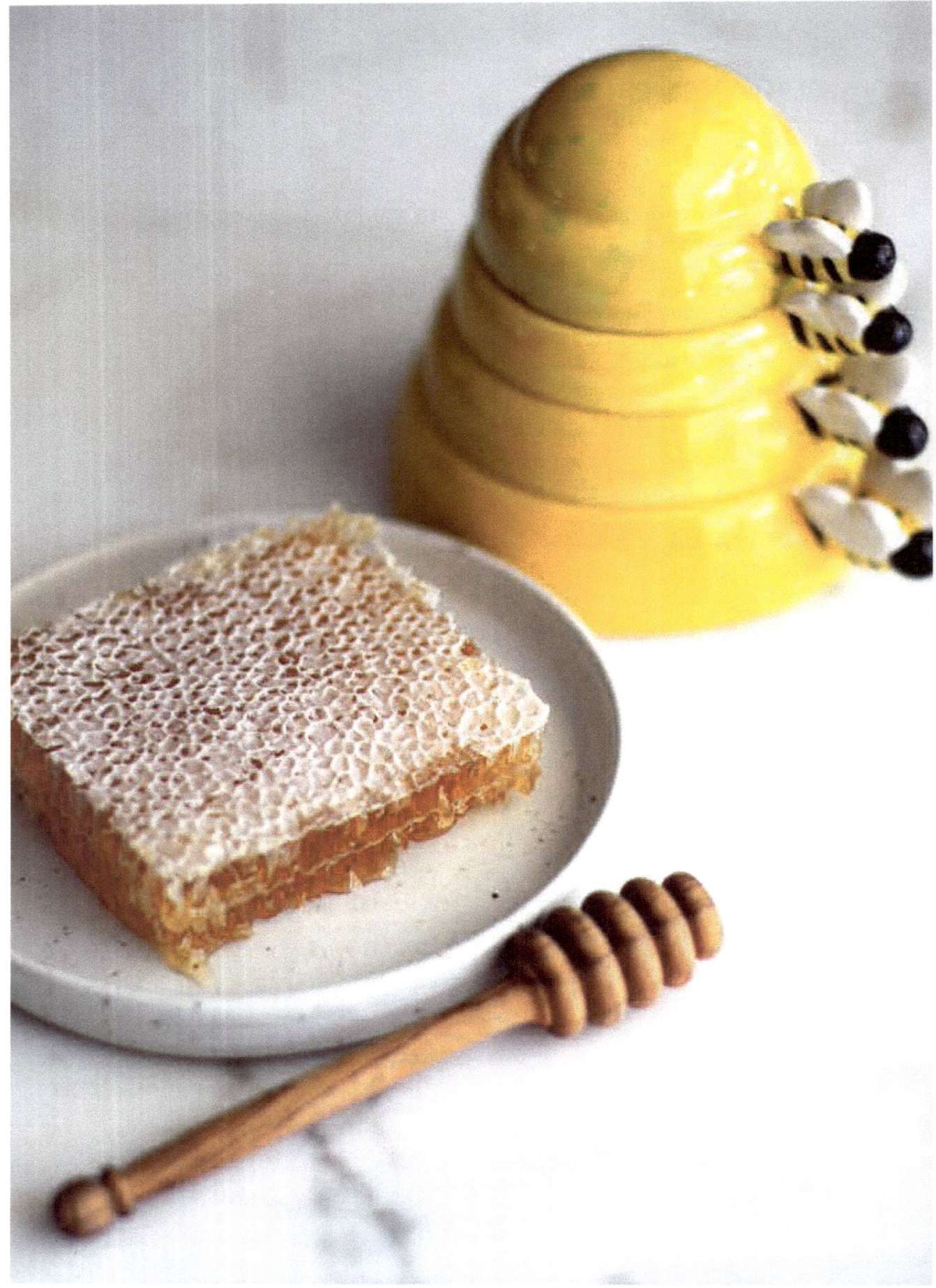

THE SWEET STUFF

MAPLE SYRUP

When I visited Canada years ago, I saw the beautiful maple trees being tapped for their syrup. The taste is unparalleled to any other sweeteners I have used (besides honey, of course). It has some good minerals in there too. Incredibly, it takes 40 litres of unrefined syrup to make just one litre of the syrup we use. I have experimented with rice malt, agave and coconut sugar but I always end up using maple and honey. But if you wish to use those too that is fine.

I intentionally choose organic maple syrup because it is farmed without chemicals and is done so very sustainably. Quality is everything, so where possible buy a really good organic Canadian maple syrup, staying away from anything that says it's "maple syrup flavoured". This usually means it's a synthetic, artificially sweetened version that is nothing like the real thing. Maple syrup generally has a slight smoky flavour to it, making such a unique addition to raw chocolate. It is still deemed a sugar with sucrose content, so the sweetness level can be reduced for people who like their cacao a little more bitter than others.

HONEY

I just love, love, love bees. Just watching their tireless efforts day in day out makes me smile, so I do all I can to help conserve and protect them.

Honey possesses anti-microbial properties. I like to look at it like a highly potent medicine that can be added to any food, snack or chocolate treat to give it a powerful boost. Honey has been found in ancient Egyptian tombs still intact, so they knew how good this stuff was too!

Honey has more fructose and glucose, and a lower sucrose content than maple syrup. It is a lot more dense than maple syrup so I have found that sometimes it can sink and separate when pouring into moulds.

Again you get what you pay for, so try to source either a local apiarist or an organic raw honey, and choose good quality honey that is free from processing as much as possible.

VANILLA

While not technically a sweetener, it does lend a note of sweetness when used in these recipes. I like to use vanilla powder if I can get it, but there was a vanilla shortage a while ago and it was hard to get powder, so I have been using vanilla paste in a tube – if you can't get either of these just use vanilla extract or essence.

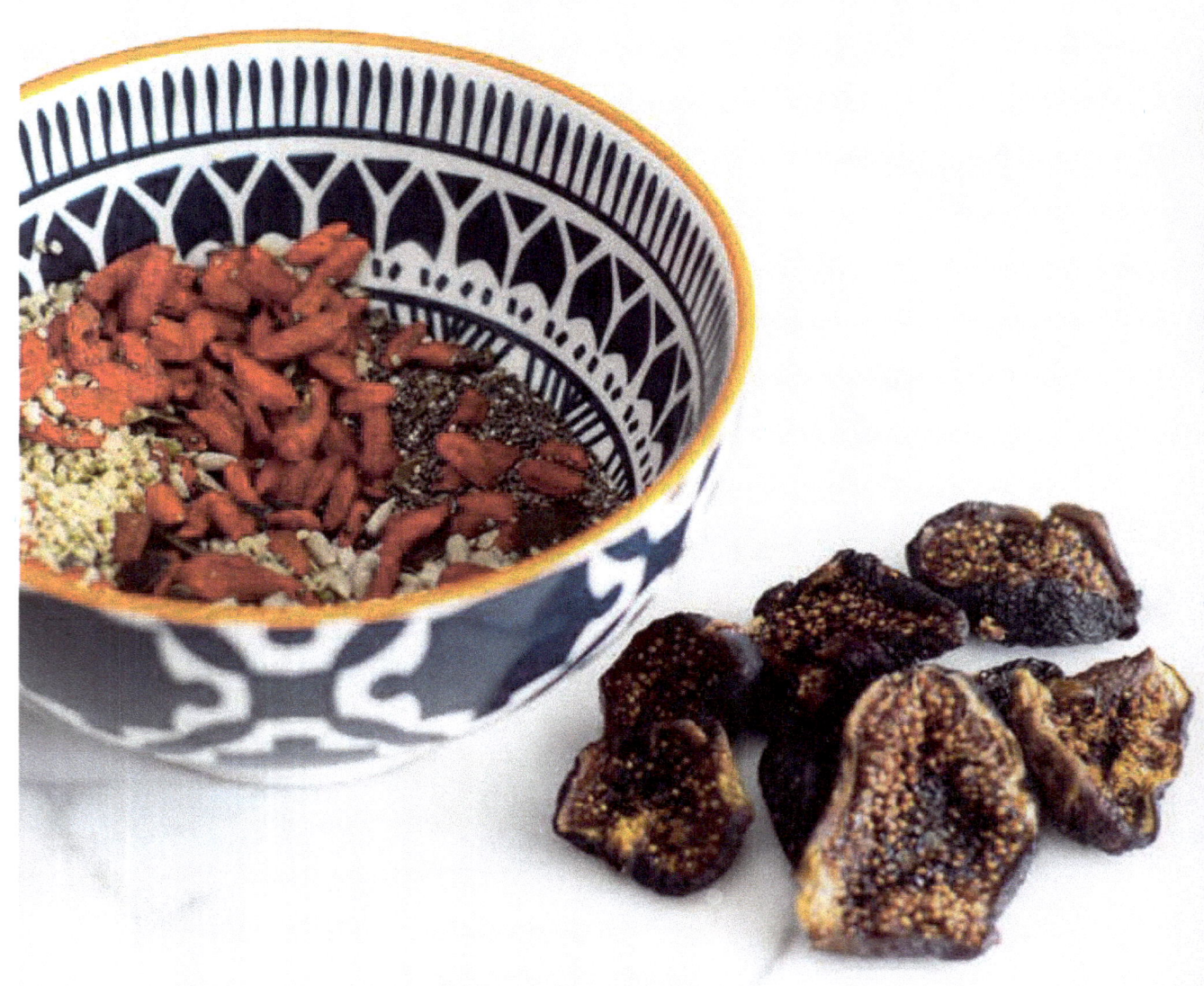

NUTS SEEDS FRUITS

CHIA SEEDS A really good source of omega 3, these little seeds are so good to add to anything and everything. They provide long lasting energy and can assist with a healthy metabolism. They can be used whole, ground or soaked for a wide variety of recipes.

DATES Medjool dates are my preference just for their sweetness, texture and flavour. I have found that with dried dates the sweetness level is quite high, the taste is very different, and the result really varies as opposed to Medjool. They make a gooey amazing raw caramel with the shredded coconut so easily and pack a punch of good sugars, fibre, and minerals.

FIGS A delicious and nutritious addition to slices, figs are packed with fibre, and minerals like magnesium, copper and vitamin B6, giving any recipe that added depth of flavour and health kick. Plus they remind me of Italy too!

GOJI BERRIES Another berry high in antioxidants, the goji is a very versatile one. I like to remove them from the fridge or the package and let them aerate for a few hours, so that they soften and are supple for eating and blending.

HEMP SEEDS A wonderful source of protein, but the best bit is they are a brain food, high in omega's that are essential for optimal health. You can whizz them up with filtered water to make Hemp milk, blitz them up to make hemp butter or just use the hulled type (that I always use) in chocolates to give that extra consistency and flavour. I even sprinkle them through salads as well.

PEPITAS A.K.A Pumpkin seeds are very high in zinc, so they are great for immune-boosting recipes. They have a nutty flavour and if you are able to source them from a good organic place, you will notice the difference – usually organic ones are double the size, flatter and a deeper green colour.

POPPY I have grown poppy plants for years and get very excited at harvest time, as the abundance of seeds that I gather is phenomenal. I add them to lots of recipes to give texture and health benefits too, with calcium, phosphorous and iron.

SESAME SEEDS Sesame seeds make a nice addition to any treat, they are high in calcium, and many other vitamins and minerals, and when roasted the flavour changes, complimenting cacao amazingly.

SUN MUSCATS I choose sun muscats for their plumpness and flavour. They complement chocolate so well and are full of goodness like B vitamins and have anti-oxidative properties too.

SUNFLOWER SEEDS A versatile seed often added to salads, smoothies and chocolates, containing good fats and oils, it has many health benefits such as supporting the thyroid with their high selenium content, and essential vitamins and minerals.

WHITE MULBERRIES These unusual berries are great in chocolates and slices due to their sharpness/sweetness of flavour. High in antioxidants, protein and fibre, they can also help support healthy cholesterol levels.

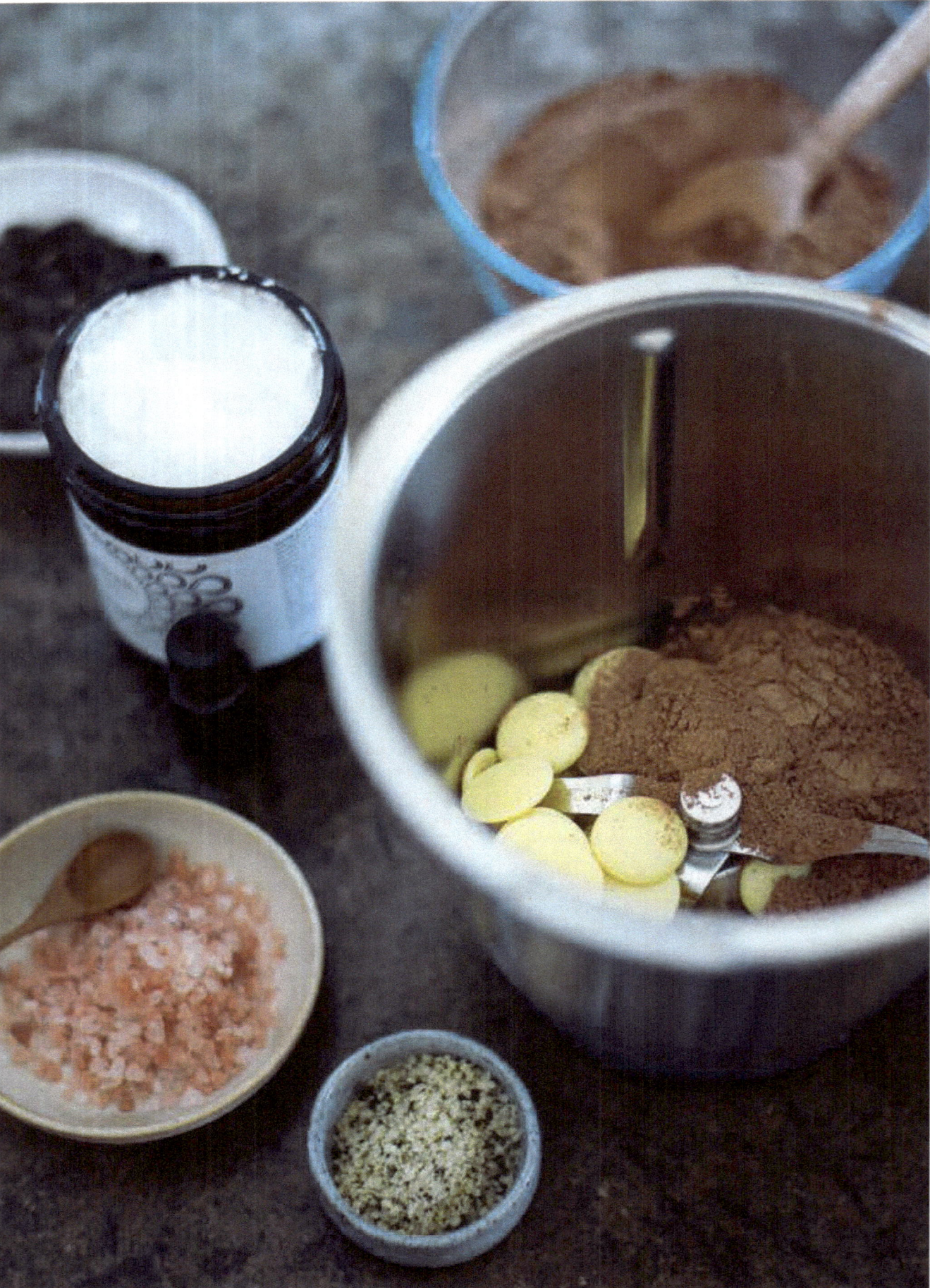

UNUSUAL INGREDIENTS

DAMIANA LEAVES I first encountered Damiana herb many years ago in a tea form. Traditionally used as an aphrodisiac, stress reliever and libido raiser, it can be drunk in a tea or ingested in foods. It has also been used to promote good digestion and just an all-round relaxant to the nervous system.

CRYSTALIZED GINGER Ginger is a great digestive aid, and a good quality dried and crystalized version has a bit of a spicy warming aftertaste to it. It's a nice surprise addition to chocolate, and compliments nuts and seeds in cacao.

BEE POLLEN These are the little clusters you see under bees' legs – it's the pollen they collect from flowers but once gathered the bees do something quite miraculous to it that changes the nutrient content of it. This is what is usually fed to the young bees as a source of food, so make sure you are getting bee pollen from a sustainable source. Bee keepers have little gatherers that gently remove the pollen once the bee is coming back to the hive, but they only do this for a short while to ensure the small bees don't go hungry or deplete stocks.

INCA BERRIES A sweet/sour sensation that I love to add to raw chocolates to contrast against the bitterness that cacao sometimes brings. Also known as a Cape Gooseberry, this is the dried version and is high in anti-oxidants, potassium, vitamins, fibre and minerals.

AMARANTH FLAKES I came across these many years back and add them to yoghurt, cacao, and other grains and seeds. They are really high in protein and many essential vitamins and are a staple of many South Americans. I have also used them in the puffed form and are delicious in slices, sprinkled on yoghurt and just to nibble on.

BUCKWHEAT Actually a rhubarb relative, buckwheat is not actually a wheat and makes a great alternative for gluten intolerant people. It has a nice nutty flavour and makes a great addition to cacao as they are super crunchy and have a powerhouse of health benefits too..

TAHINI A regular addition to many recipes, it is a paste made from ground sesame seeds that is super high in calcium and many vitamins and minerals. It's also delicious added to slices or soft centre chocolates to give a deeper, intense sesame flavour.

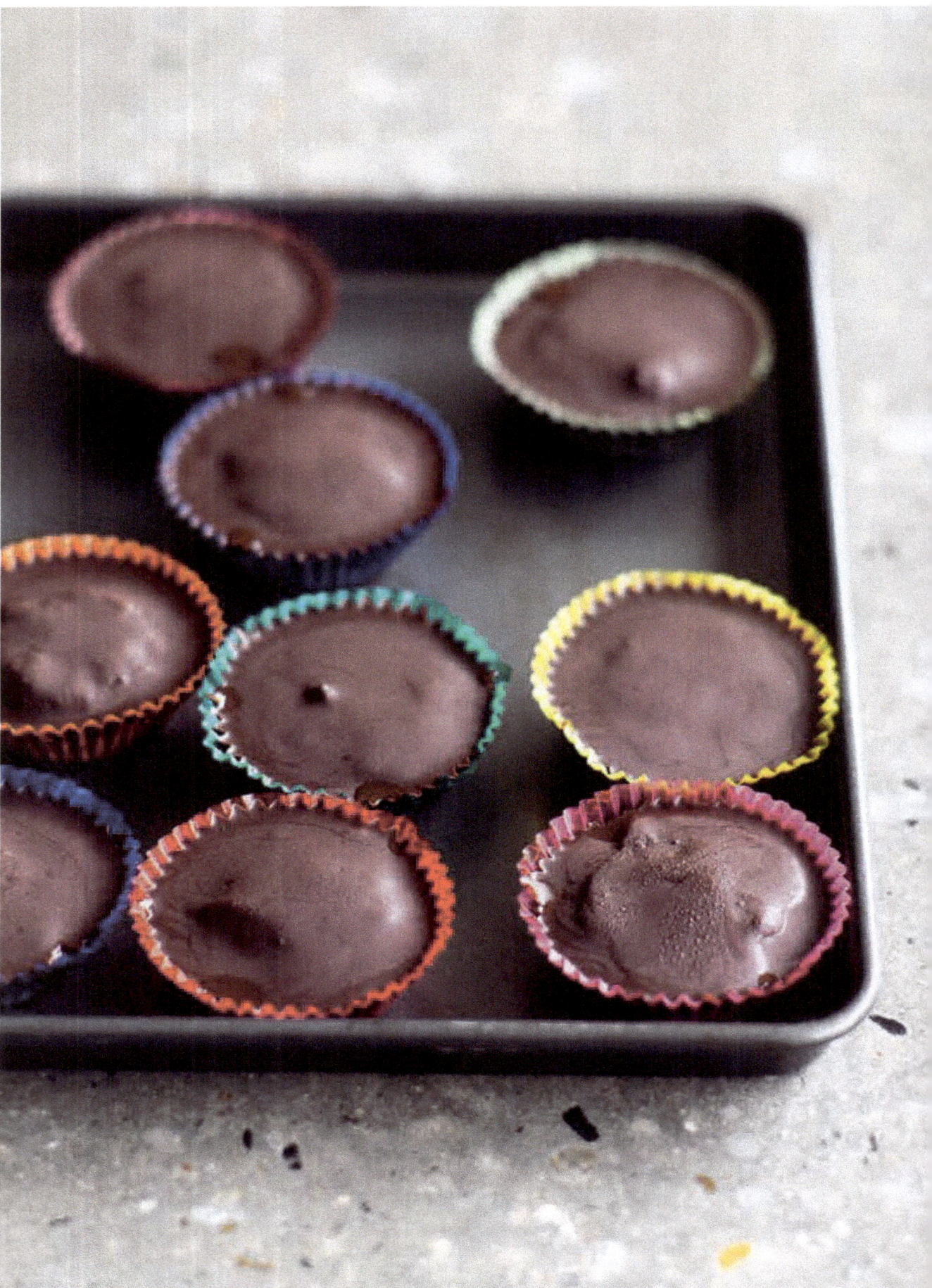

NOTES, TIPS AND TRICKS

THERMOMIX
Where possible, recipes in CacaoAddict include a set of instructions for those cacao lovers who have a Thermomix – these are denoted by a **TM** in the instructions. Those who don't use a Thermomix can simply ignore these instructions. The gram weight indicated in the ingredients lists is there for Thermomix users or those who like to weigh rather than measure.

DOUBLE BOILER
Melting ingredients using a double boiler method allows for easier control of the process, as you can see the ingredients change and will know when to pull it off the heat.

Simply place 1 to 2 cups of water in a small to medium sized saucepan and bring to a simmer. Place a heatproof bowl on top of your saucepan with the ingredients you need to melt (in this book, usually coconut oil and cacao butter). Stir as they melt. Once they have combined, add the rest of the chocolate ingredients and mix well until they are all combined and have a nice glossy finish.

TIP Keep any water out of making hard chocolates, as it throws the mixture out. Pay attention if you are making chocolates using a double boiler method for melting as water can easily sneak in.

TRAYS AND PANS
You don't need too many different trays for this book. For recipes using patty pans, I just line the pans up on a metal baking tray. For the balls or bark recipes, I generally use a medium sized flat baking tray lined with greaseproof paper, and for the fudges and thicker slabs I use a medium rectangular silicon form, or a greaseproof paper lined small baking dish.

MAKES
I haven't noted how many serves these recipes create as it depends very much on how large you might crack the bark, how big you roll a ball, how small you chop a fudge and so on. Rest assured that each recipe will nourish you and your friends, and you might even have some left over for tomorrow (again, that depends on you!).

SALT
I have indicated to use pink, also known as Himalayan, salt in these recipes. Pink salt gets its lovely rosy colour from trace minerals such as magnesium, potassium and calcium, and is usually less processed than other table salt. Celtic sea salt is another good alternative.

ESSENTIAL OILS
When adding essential oils into food always look at what you are doing. Some oils are more viscous than others and particularly with stronger flavour oils, less is best. Add the oils into a fat, either coconut oil or melted cacao butter, otherwise if a drop falls onto a nut or a seed the taste can be very intense, rather than be distributed through the whole recipe.

SOAKING BERRIES
Goji berries can tend to be quite hard and sharp, but have found if I leave them out in a bowl 1-2 hours before using them it changes the consistency to soft and chewy. They will blend easier too.

MELT DOWN
Always keep your cacao creations in the fridge after you have made them. They will keep for around two weeks in an airtight container, and will freeze for a few months if need be.

Unless indicated, enjoy your treats straight from the fridge, as sitting too long at room temperature could result in some loss of form.

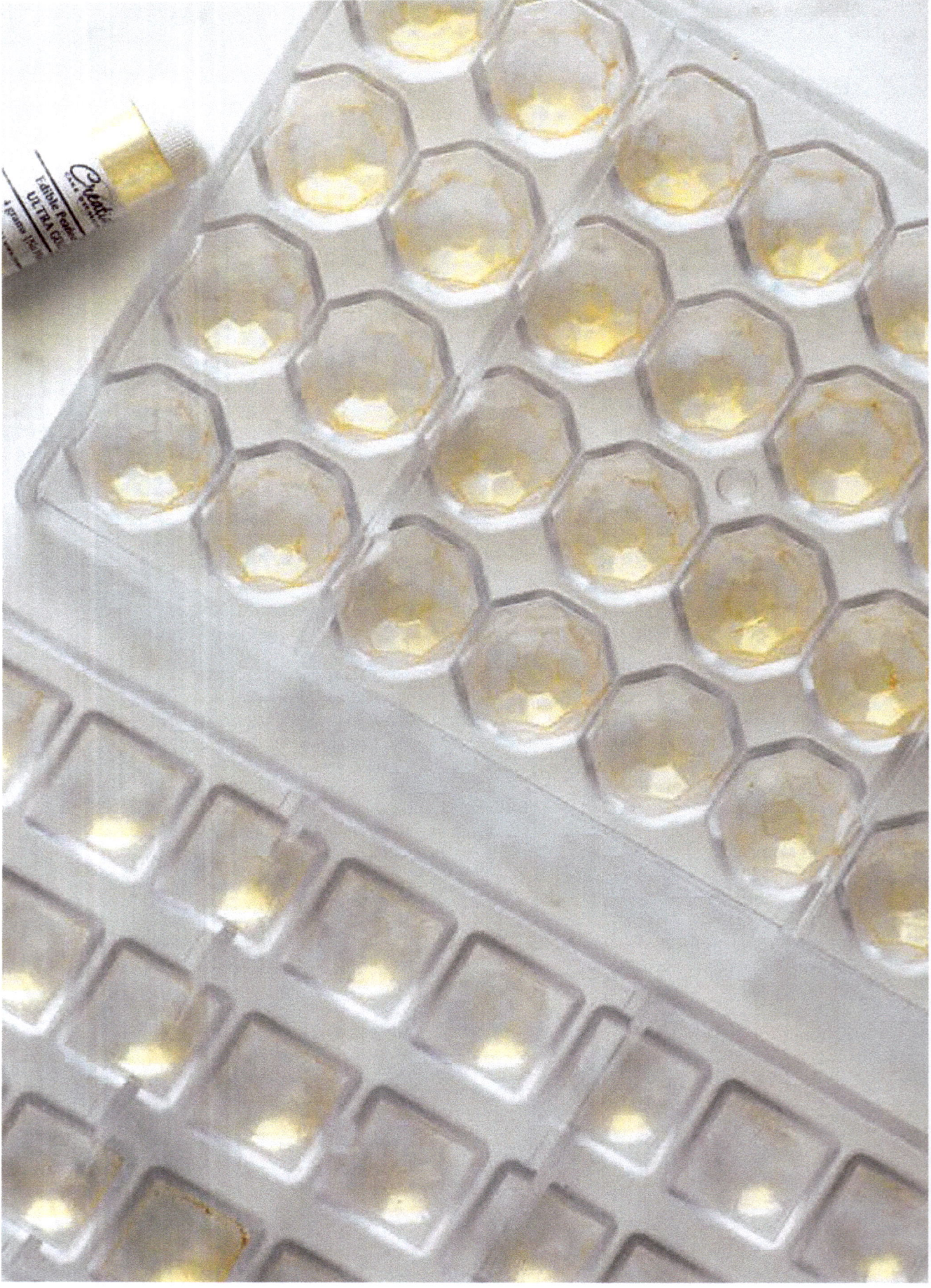

KNOW YOUR MOULDS

You can buy chocolate moulds easily these days, however the quality and price can range widely.

SILICON Make sure you get decent quality silicon. When using, remember that they are bendy so need to be placed onto a board or a tray before filling and transporting to the fridge. They are easy to push out when they are set as you can press them from the bottom and the little chocolates just come out.

HARD PLASTIC You can pay up to $30 a tray for good quality European professional moulds and the results are stunning. The chocolates tend to take longer to set in these compared to silicon, and to get the chocolates out its also an art that requires practice. Turn them upside down and evenly in a smooth quick fashion, banging onto a chopping board, and repeating until they all come out. The sheen and shine of these moulds are next level and you can also use edible dusts in these moulds for a glossy and glitzy finish.

TIP When filling the chocolate moulds you don't have to be too precise with filling each hole separately, instead pour the chocolate over the whole mould tray and scrape the excess into your Thermomix or a bowl with a silicon spatula or metal scraper.

ACTIVATED NUTS

Activated nuts are nuts that have been soaked for a period of time (usually 7-12 hours) before they are dried out on low heat in an oven or dehydrator (around 65°C for 12-24 hours). This stimulates the germination and sprouting process of the nut, which increases the bioavailability of nutrients and makes them more digestible by breaking down the enzymes which we find hard to deal with.

Buying nuts already activated certainly will save you some time and effort, but they are more costly. If you can get in the habit of doing it yourself at home, you will always have jars of activated nuts ready to snack on and use in these recipes. Note that home-activated nuts can be prone to mould so they need to be eaten within a couple of days. Keeping them in the fridge in an airtight jar helps keep them fresh.

HOW TO Place nuts in a large bowl and cover with filtered water. The nuts should be completely covered. Add approximately ½ to 1 teaspoon of sea salt to one cup of almonds, and soak for 7-12 hours.

Drain off excess water. Place nuts on a baking tray and dry out on your oven's lowest heat setting (around 65°C) for 12-24 hours. They are ready when completely dried out. (sometimes without doing the whole drying process, I still love to soak almonds overnight with the salt and water, and then drain and use them in some recipes, I leave them out for about an hour or two on a clean tea towel just to aerate and dry slightly, you are still getting the nutritional benefits, plus removing most of those enzymes and tannins)

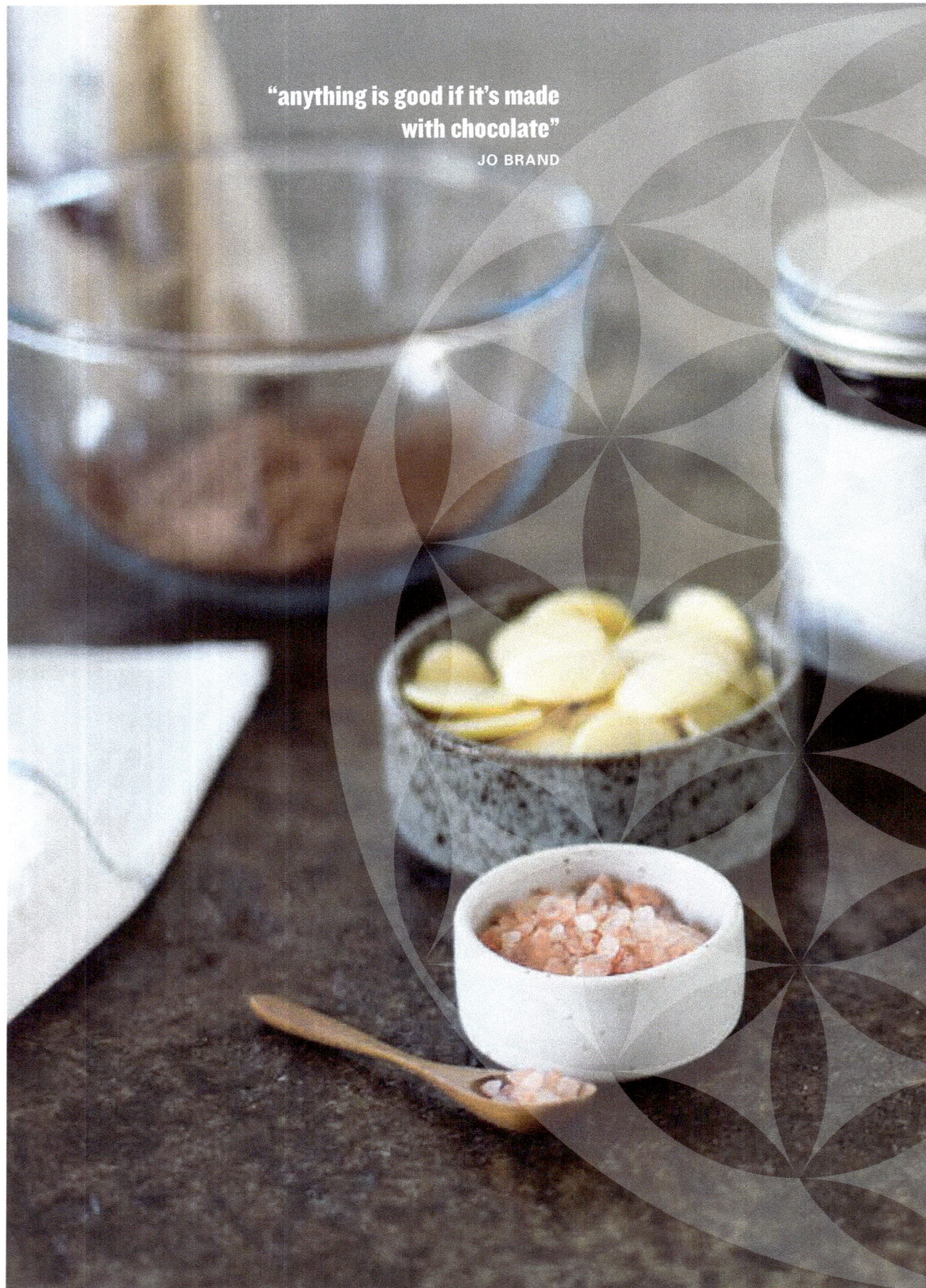

"anything is good if it's made with chocolate"
JO BRAND

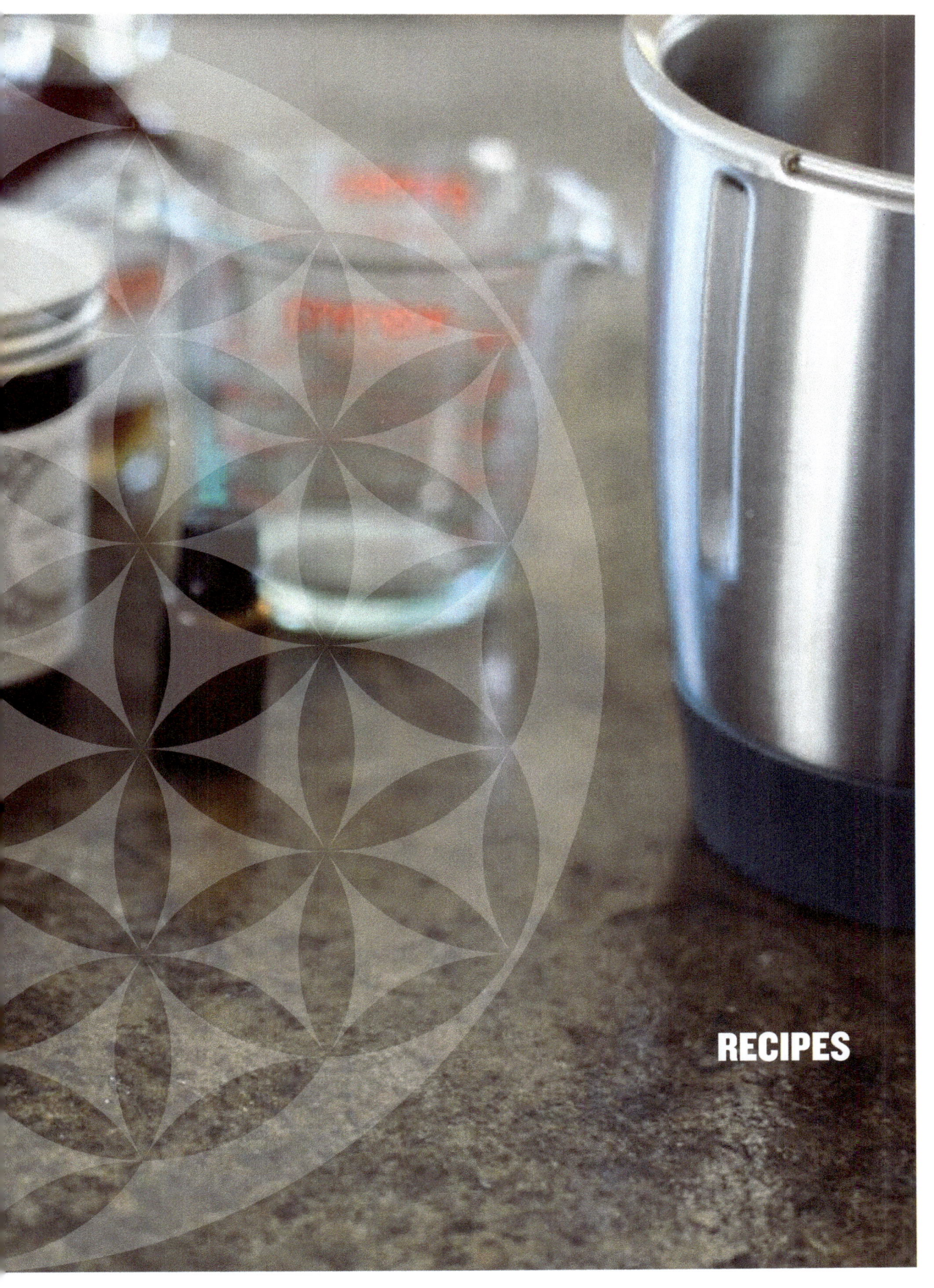

RECIPES

Basic chocolate recipe

My fool-proof chocolate recipe that can be used as a base to add any nuts, seeds, grains, superfood powders and food-grade essential oils into. This makes a hard-snap set chocolate.

Melt cacao butter and coconut oil first on low heat (**TM** heat 50, speed 2, 5 minutes) or using the double boiler method (see below). Then add in cacao powder, maple syrup and salt, mixing well to form a smooth glossy batter. The longer you mix, the better the chocolate flavour, texture and consistency.

TIP Any addition of superfood powders will thicken the mix slightly.

DOUBLE BOILER METHOD
Simply place 1 to 2 cups of water in a small to medium sized saucepan and bring to a simmer.

Place a heatproof bowl on top of your saucepan with the coconut oil and cacao butter. Stir as they melt.

Once they have combined, add the rest of the chocolate ingredients and mix well until they are all combined and have a nice glossy finish.

---

1 cup (120g) cacao butter

¼ cup (45g) coconut oil

1 cup (100g) organic cacao powder

¼ cup (70g) maple syrup

Pinch of pink salt

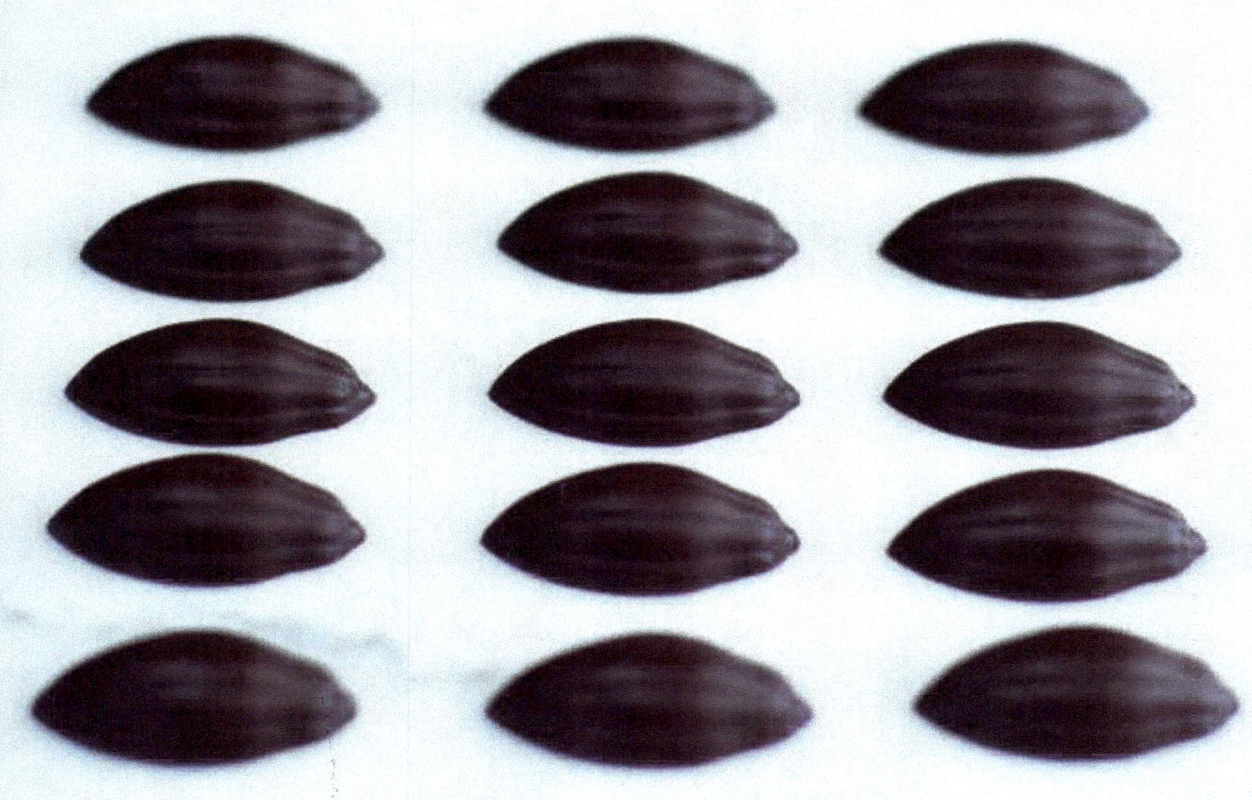

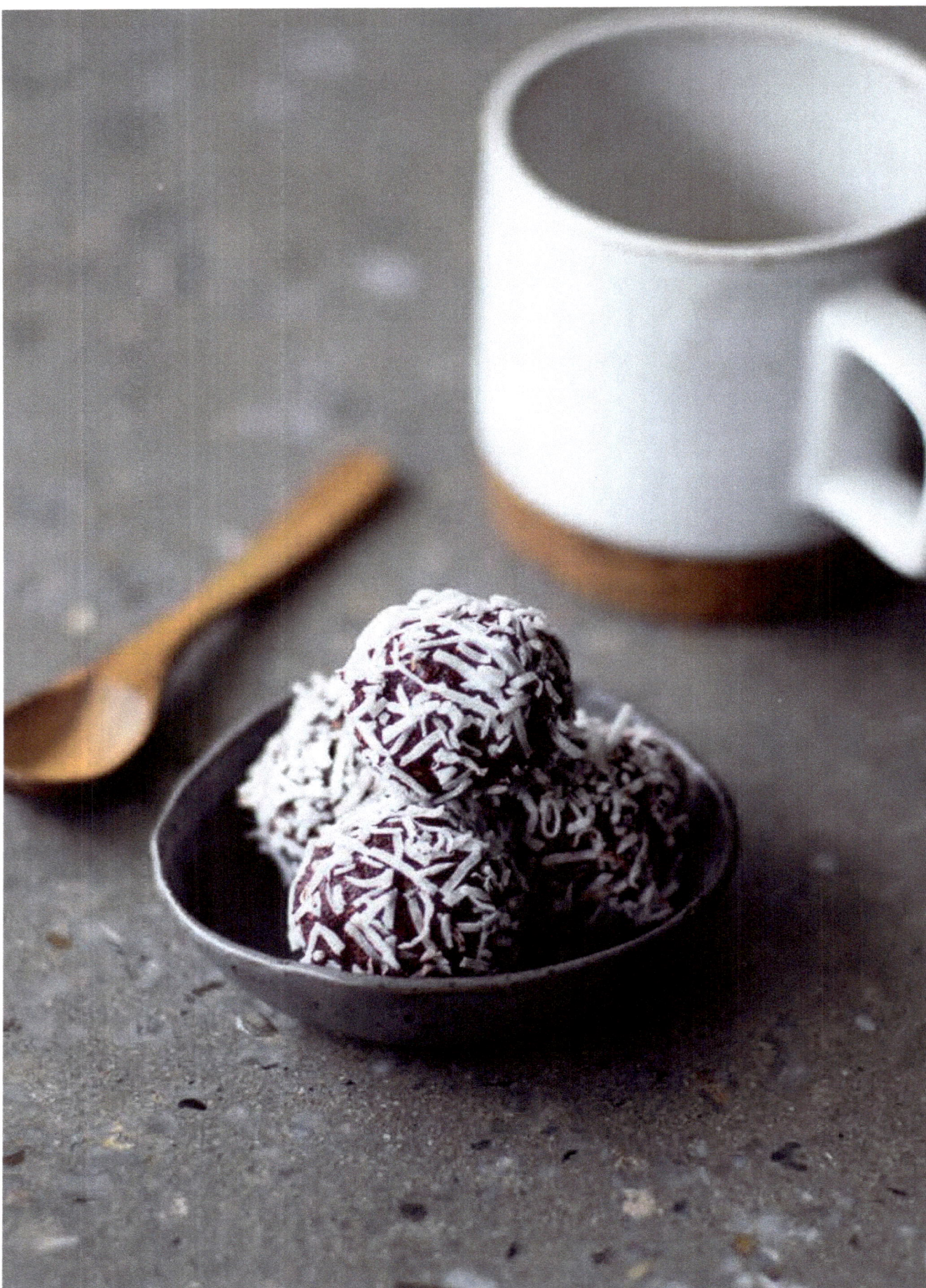

Red Velvet Cardamom Truffles

With the healing colour and texture of beetroot, these truffles are not just medicine for the body but also food for the soul. They are simple to make, and there is something quite satisfying about knowing you are eating chocolate with your vegetables!

Place all ingredients into your food processor or Thermomix. Blend at high speed (**TM** 7 through 9) until the mixture is smooth, well-combined and sticking together. It should be a beautiful red, velvety texture. If you want it sweeter, add another tablespoon of maple syrup.

Use your hands to shape the mixture into bite-size balls, then roll the balls with the extra shredded coconut and place in the fridge to set, it should take around one hour. Allow the balls to come to room temperature 10 minutes before serving.

TIP To allow the balls to roll easily without sticking, wear a pair of disposable gloves rubbed with just a touch of coconut oil.

1 small beetroot, quartered then parboiled
1¼ cups (100g) shredded coconut, plus extra for rolling
12 Medjool dates, pitted
½ cup (65g) almonds
5 tbsp (35g) organic cacao powder
3 tbsp (50g) maple syrup
4 drops food-grade cardamom essential oil
10 drops food-grade wild orange essential oil
½ tsp vanilla paste
Pinch of pink salt

Pure Rose Oil Cacao

Rose has always been a symbol of love, purity and connection to me, so when I was able to source a pure Bulgarian rose essential oil to add into chocolate, I knew it would be next level stuff. These always come out when I have a special occasion to celebrate – everyone just feels so open hearted and warm when savoring them.

Using the double boiler method, place the cacao butter and coconut oil together in a heat-proof bowl, and set this over a small saucepan of simmering water (**TM** heat 50, speed 2, 5 minutes). Stir together as they melt, then mix in the remaining ingredients to form a rich chocolate batter (**TM** speed 3, 4 minutes). Pour the mixture into chocolate moulds and refrigerate until set, approximately one hour.

Eat with reverence and an open heart.

- 1 cup (120g) cacao butter
- 1 cup (100g) organic cacao powder
- ¼ cup (45g) coconut oil
- ¼ cup (70g) maple syrup
- 1 tsp maca powder
- 1 drop food-grade rose essential oil
- Pinch of pink salt

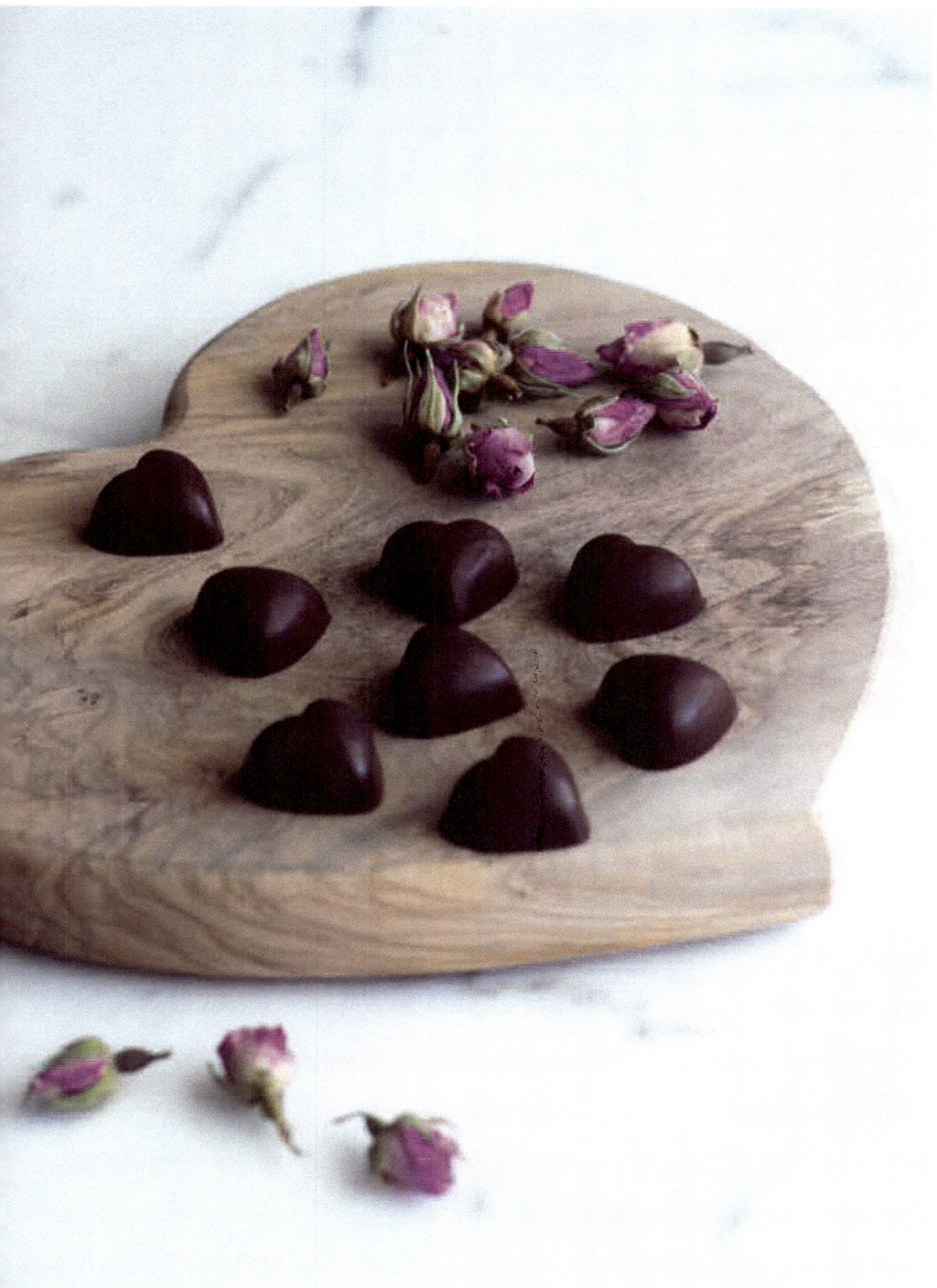

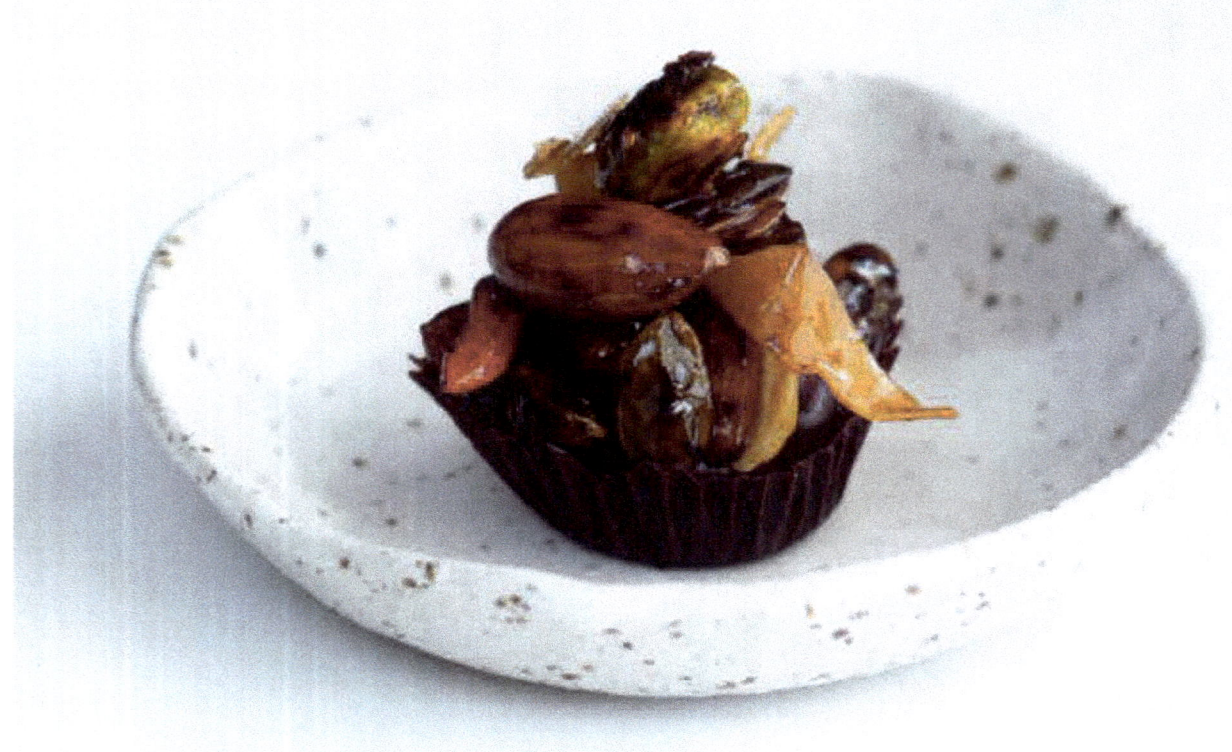

Roasted Nuts in Raw Chocolate Ginger Cups

Food for me is often like art – a balance of sensory elements and a whole-body experience. The sharp, warming ginger notes combined with the visual toppings and multiple flavour and texture sensations mean that these cups are often requested and always loved.

Set roughly 20 paper patty pans on a baking tray. Place a frying pan over medium heat, and toast the nuts, pepitas, goji berries and coconut, stirring constantly. Do each separately as they toast at different rates. Set aside together in a bowl to cool.

In double boiler, melt cacao butter and coconut oil over low heat (**TM** heat 50, speed 2, 5 minutes). Add the cacao powder, maple syrup, ginger oil, vanilla paste and salt and mix well. Spoon a tablespoon of this mixture into each patty pan.

When the frying pan is cooler, place over low heat and put the nut filling mixture back in the pan and add the honey. Stir, allowing it to bubble into a toffee. Place a spoonful of nut mix on top of each chocolate cup and refrigerate for one hour.

NOTES If you have extra of the chocolate mixture you can drizzle over top of the nuts before refrigerating.

CUPS
- 1 cup (120g) cacao butter
- ⅓ cup (60g) coconut oil
- 1 cup (100g) organic cacao powder
- ¼ cup (70g) of maple syrup
- 1 tsp vanilla paste
- 6 drops food-grade ginger essential oil
- Pinch of pink salt

NUT FILLING
- 1 cup (130g) pistachio nuts
- 1 cup (130g) activated almonds
- 1 cup (130g) pepitas
- ½ cup (60g) goji berries
- ½ cup (30g) shredded coconut
- ½ cup (150g) honey

Cashew Lime Cups

Cashews are such a good friend to have in the kitchen. These versatile nuts can be soaked, toasted, used either as savoury or sweet, and their texture can morph into a range of useful applications. I use them in three layer centres and as a soft centre base to lots of my creations.

Set roughly 20 paper patty pans on a baking tray. First, make the cacao base. Using the double boiler method over low heat, melt cacao butter and coconut oil and add in cacao powder, maple syrup, salt and mix well (**TM** heat 50, speed 2, 5 minutes). Spoon into patty tins and spread up the sides of each patty pan, and refrigerate for about 10 minutes or until set. Remove from fridge, then repeat with a small amount of chocolate mixture up the sides to strengthen the cup. Return the tray to the refrigerator to set.

Drain cashews and place in a food processor or Thermomix, with blueberries, tahini and maple syrup. Blend (**TM** speed 4), scraping down sides a few times, adding one tablespoon of coconut water at a time until the consistency forms a smooth cream. Spoon cream into chocolate cups and sprinkle with toasted coconut and nibs.

CACAO BASE

1 cup (120g) cacao butter

¼ cup (45g) coconut oil

1 cup (100g) organic cacao powder

¼ cup (70g) maple syrup

Pinch of pink salt

CASHEW FILLING

1 cup (130g) cashews, soaked overnight in springwater

½ cup (60g) blueberries

1 tbsp tahini

2 tbsp maple syrup

1 tbsp coconut oil

Approx 100ml coconut water (amount will vary depending on your cashews)

1 tsp almond butter

½ tsp vanilla paste

4 drops of food-grade lime essential oil

1 tbsp cacao nibs

¼ cup (15g) toasted coconut

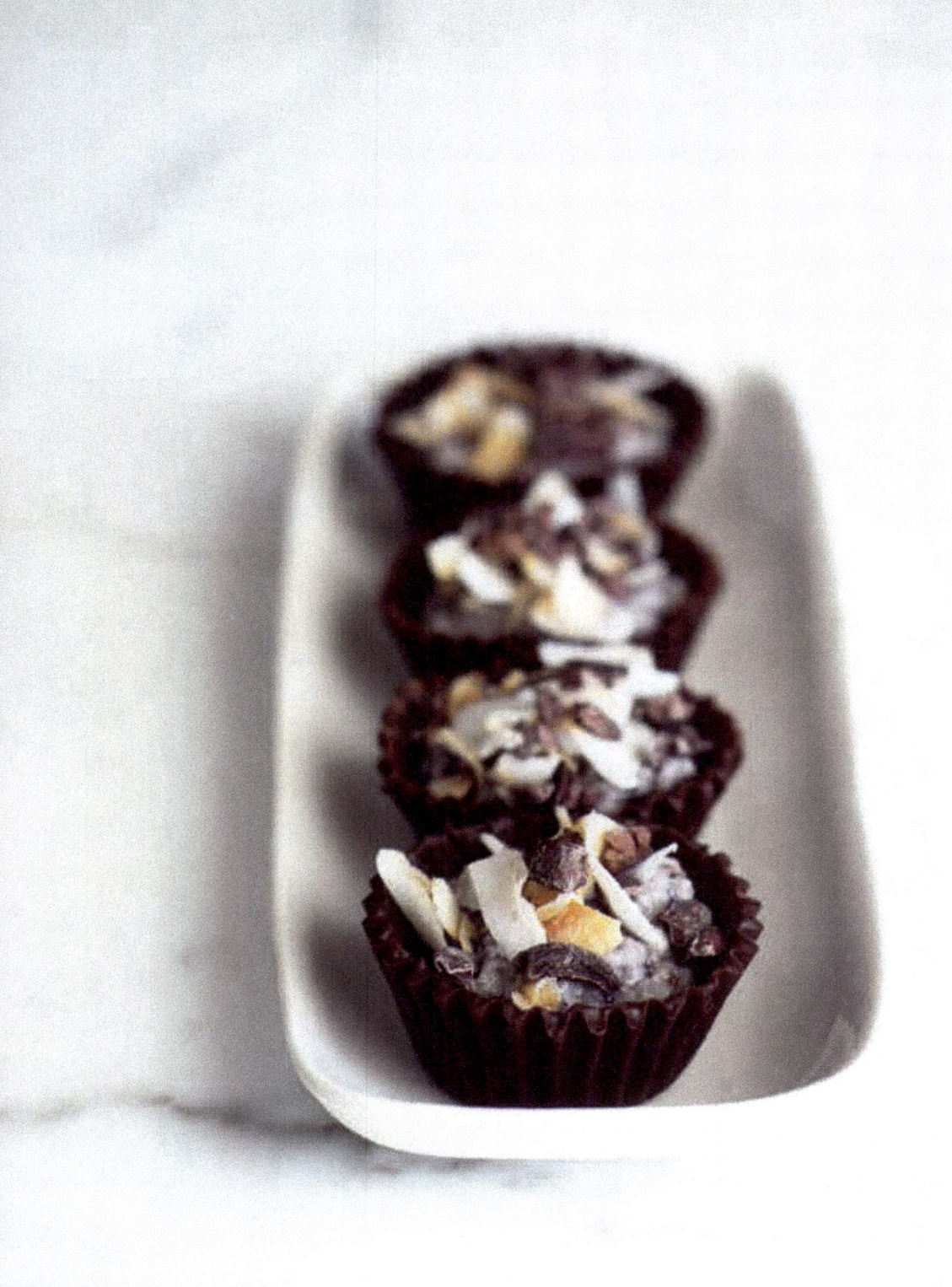

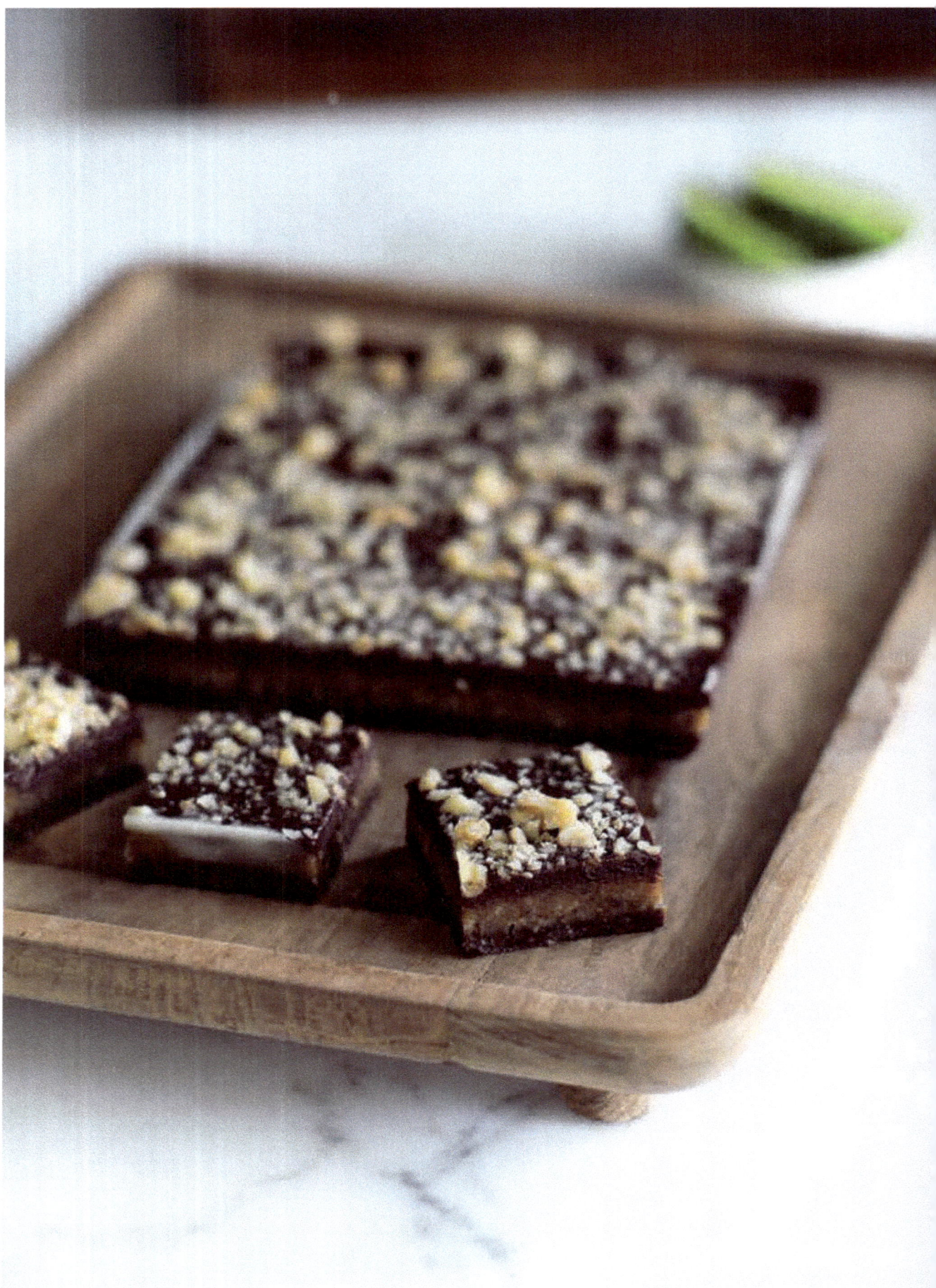

Triple Layer Ginger and Lime Caramel Slice

There is something about a layered treat that really feels exciting and decadent. But unlike most OTT desserts, this slice contains plant-based proteins, superfoods and nutrient-dense foods, so you will feel satisfied for hours.

Use either a rectangular silicone form, or line a small ceramic baking dish with greaseproof paper. Make the base first by pulsing dates, almonds, coconut oil, hemp protein, cacao, honey and ginger oil in a food processor until it forms a crumble (**TM** speed 8, 40 seconds).

Press this mixture into the slice tin, pressing down until firm and smooth. Place in the freezer while you create the middle layer.

To make the caramel-walnut layer, place dates, coconut oil, tahini, vanilla and honey in a food processor. Process until smooth (**TM** Speed 7, 30 seconds, scraping down sides until smooth).

Pour the caramel-walnut mixture on top of the base, smooth out and return to freezer for approximately 15 minutes until partially set.

Mix together the melted coconut oil, raw cacao and maple syrup in a bowl until smooth.

Once the caramel-walnut layer is partially set, remove from the freezer and spread the chocolate layer on top, then sprinkle over the chopped walnuts.

Return to the freezer until set (about an hour), then slice into portions.

NOTES If the middle layer is too cold when you are ready to add the top ganache layer, the ganache will set too quickly, and thus affect the consistency of this layer. I suggest you work quickly to spread the ganache to avoid this.

BASE

7 Medjool dates, pitted
½ cup (65g) activated almonds
3 tbsp (20g) raw organic cacao powder
2 tbsp coconut oil
2 tbsp (60g) raw honey
1 tbsp hemp protein powder
5 drops of food-grade ginger essential oil

CARAMEL WALNUT LAYER

14 Medjool dates, pitted
½ cup (90g) coconut oil
¼ cup (30g) chopped walnuts
3 tbsp (60g) tahini
1 tsp vanilla paste
2 tbsp raw honey
1 tbsp maca powder
10 drops of food-grade lime essential oil

TOP LAYER (GANACHE)

¼ cup (45g) coconut oil, melted
⅓ cup (95g) maple syrup
⅓ cup (35g) raw organic cacao powder
¼ cup (30g) chopped walnuts
1 tbsp poppy seeds
Pinch of pink salt

Buckini Nut Crunchy Cacao Slab

Buckwheat is a new addition to many recipes and unlike its name indicates, is not a grain at all, but rather a relative of rhubarb. This gluten-free seed is chock-full of important nutrients such as magnesium and B vitamins, and is also a good source of fibre. This slab combines chocolate with a peppermint blast and some pretty powerful medicinal mushroom powder, all together providing you with a multitude of health benefits.

Line a baking tray with greaseproof paper. Melt the cacao butter and coconut oil together using the double boiler method over low heat (**TM** heat 50, speed 2, 5 minutes), then add all other ingredients and mix well (don't chop if you are using a Thermomix as those Brazil nuts look so appealing when the slice is cut).

Spread mixture evenly on the baking tray, sprinkle with coconut flakes and refrigerate until set, around one hour. Cut into squares and serve.

1 cup (120g) cacao butter
⅓ cup (60g) coconut oil
1 cup (100g) organic cacao powder
1 tsp pink salt
¼ cup (70g) maple syrup
½ cup (30g) shredded coconut
¼ cup (35g) dried white mulberries
⅓ cup (55g) activated buckinis
⅓ cup (45g) Brazil nuts
1 tbsp medicinal mushroom powder
7 drops food-grade peppermint essential oil
5 drops food-grade black pepper essential oil
Coconut flakes for topping

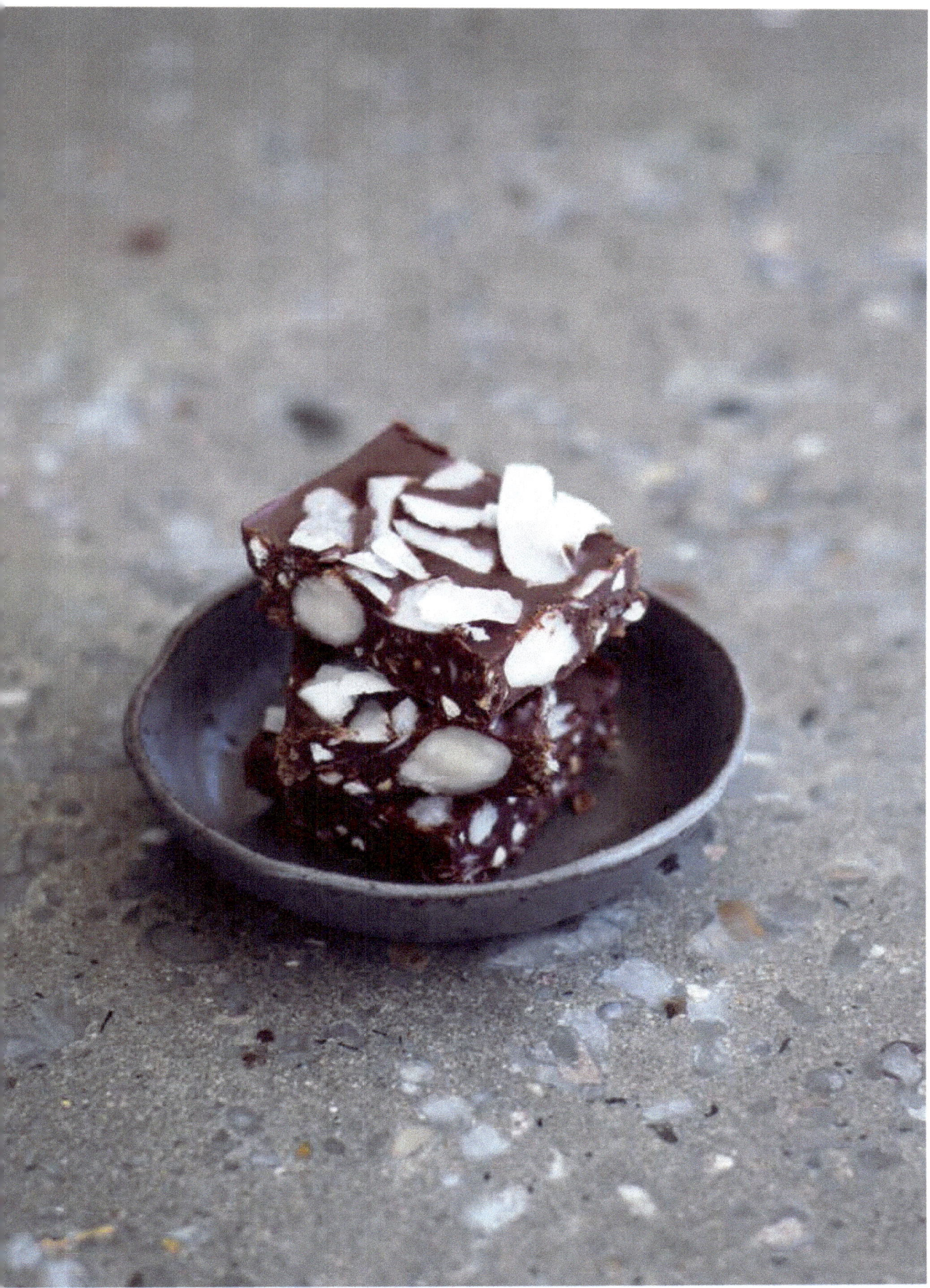

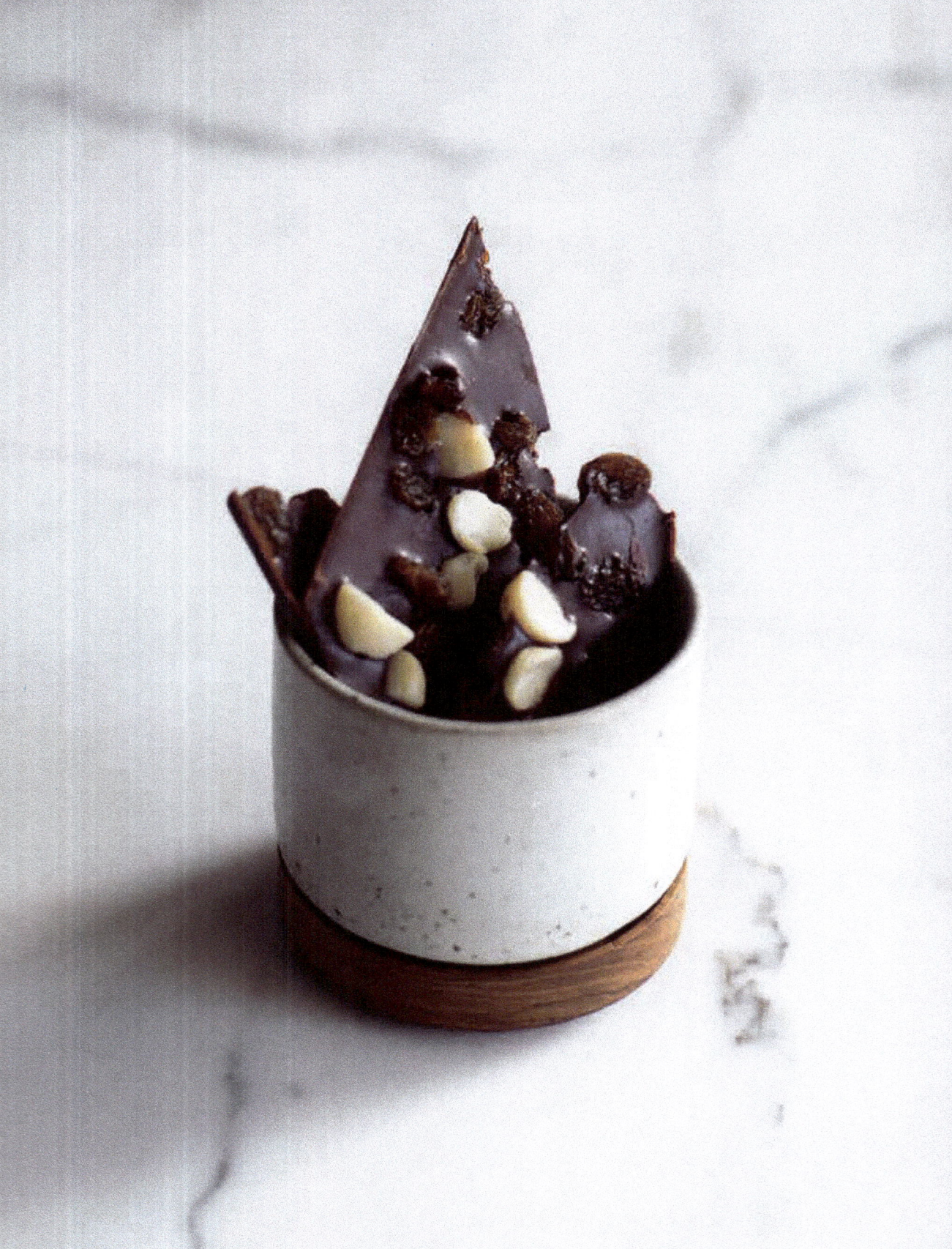

Macadamia and Muscat Bark

This bark is a lovely contradiction in flavours. Imagine the sharpness of dark cacao melting on your tongue with the creamy crunch of macadamias and the dense, sweet chewiness of sun muscat raisins... makes me want to go make some right now! I use a metabolic blend oil, which contains grapefruit, peppermint, cinnamon, ginger and lemon to help promote a healthy metabolism. It's a win all round.

Line a medium-sized baking tray with greaseproof paper. Using the double boiler method over a low heat, melt the coconut oil and cacao powder together (**TM** heat 50, speed 2, z5 minutes), and then add in powders, maple syrup, essential oil and salt and mix well.

Pour chocolate mixture onto the tray and spread out evenly. Then arrange the muscats and macadamia nuts across the surface and refrigerate for approximately one hour or until set.

Crack into pieces when serving.

1 cup (120g) cacao butter
¼ cup (45g) coconut oil
¾ cup (75g) organic cacao powder
¼ cup (70g) maple syrup
1 tsp camu camu powder
8 drops of food-grade "metabolic blend" essential oil
Pinch of pink salt
1 cup (130g) macadamia nuts
1 cup (160g) sun muscat raisins

Lime and Orange Slice

Another triple layer favourite, this time with an uplifting citrus twist. The centre layer also includes the superfood powder maca, which is a root vegetable known for its ability to help boost energy, improve stamina, assist with cognitive function, supply iron to red blood cells and loads more benefits.

Line a medium-sized baking tray with greaseproof paper. Place all of the base ingredients into a food processor or Thermomix, and blend until the mixture comes together (**TM** speed 10 for 1 minute, scrape down sides and repeat if needed). Tip mixture into the baking tray and smooth out using greaseproof paper (see notes below), then press down firmly with the back of a spoon.

Drain the cashews, and place in the food processor or Thermomix. Blend slowly (**TM** speed 4), and slowly add other ingredients until well combined. Pour over the base layer then put into the freezer for a few minutes.

Now make the top layer. Using a double boiler or a heat-proof bowl set over a saucepan of simmering water, melt cacao butter and coconut oil together (**TM** heat 50, speed 2, 5 minutes) before adding cacao powder, maple syrup and salt. Mix well.

Remove the tray from the freezer and spread the chocolate mixture over the top for your final layer. Return to freezer to set for one hour.

Once set, remove from freezer and cut into squares.

NOTES To smooth out the base, scrunch up some greaseproof paper and apply a little coconut oil, then press out the base mixture roughly over surface of tray, then smooth out with the back of a tablespoon until it's compressed and even.

BASE
1¾ cups (120g) shredded coconut
1½ cups (195g) walnuts
6 Medjool dates, pitted
3 tbsp (50g) maple syrup
3 tbsp (20g) organic cacao powder
2 tbsp coconut oil
8 drops food-grade wild orange essential oil
Pinch of pink salt

MIDDLE
1¼ cup (160g) cashews (soaked for a few hours or overnight)
4 tbsp (60g) coconut oil
5 tbsp (70g) maple syrup
1 tsp vanilla paste
1 tsp maca powder
Pinch of pink salt
12 drops of food-grade lime essential oil

TOP
2 tbsp cacao butter
2 tbsp coconut oil
¼ cup (25g) organic cacao powder
2 tbsp maple syrup
Pinch of pink salt

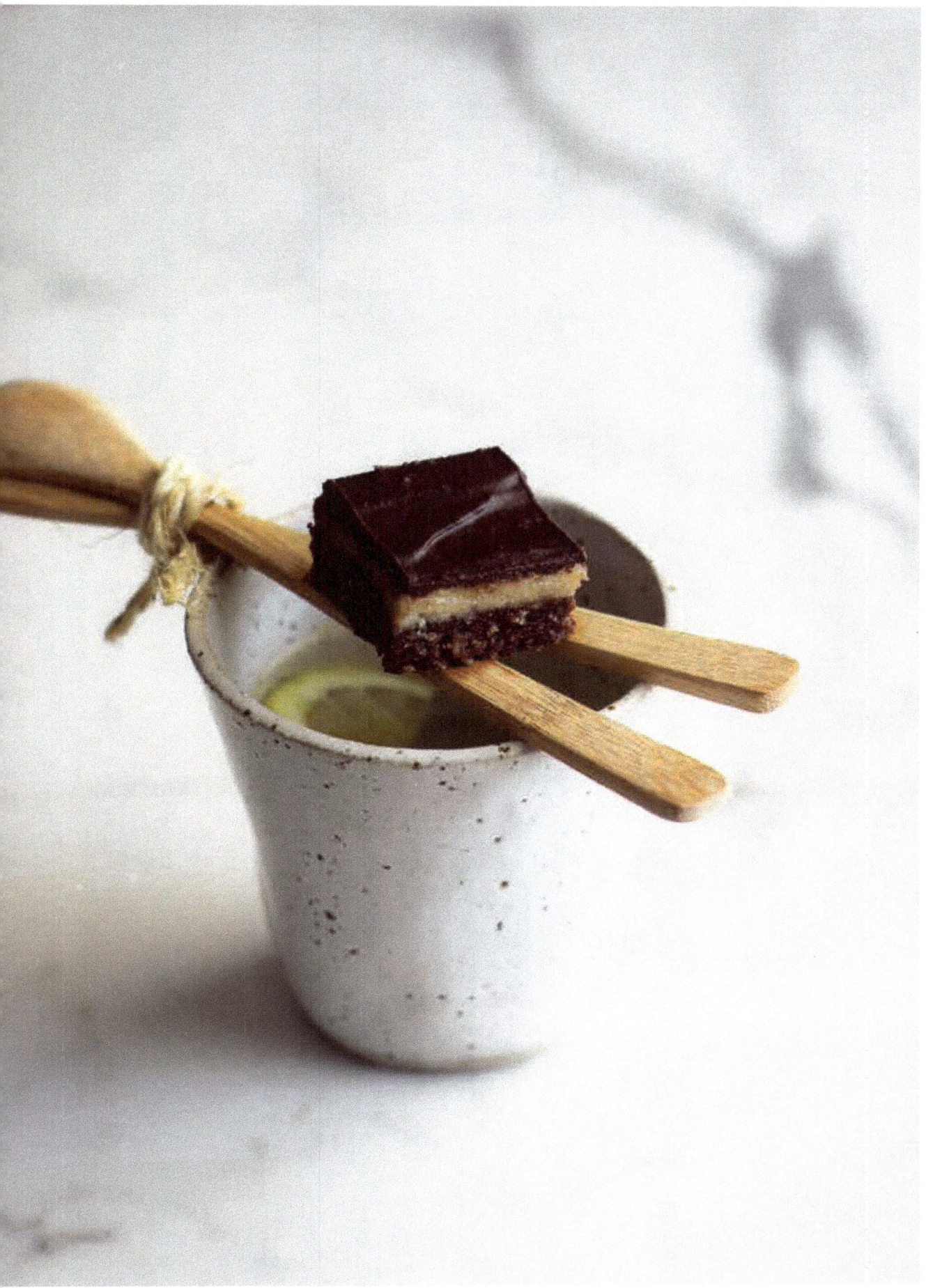

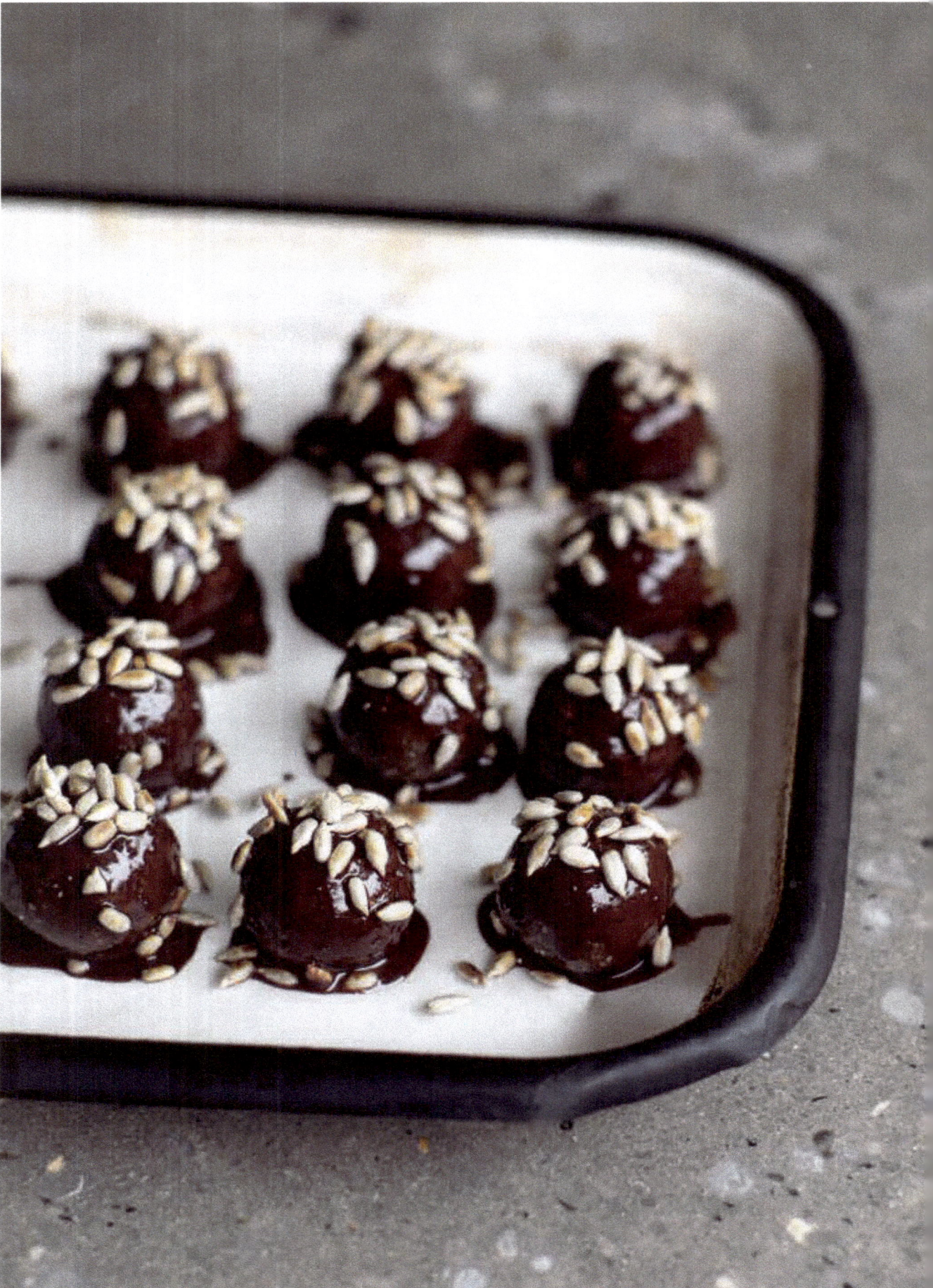

Chocolate Coated Nutty Tangerine Balls

I've always loved how seeds and nuts deliver such a dense nutrient hit with healthy fats and protein, and when combined with tangerine, chocolate and honey it takes the flavour and benefits to a whole other level.

Line a baking tray with greaseproof paper. In a small frypan over medium heat, toast the sunflower seeds with a pinch of salt, stirring continuously. Set aside to cool.

Place all ingredients except for the toasted sunflower seeds into a food processor or Thermomix. Lightly blend everything well together until it binds (**TM** speed 6, 30 seconds, scrape down sides). Take a tablespoon of mixture and roll into small balls, place on tray and refrigerate.

Using the double boiler method over low heat, melt cacao butter and coconut oil together (**TM** heat 50, speed 2, 5 minutes), then add other ingredients and mix well.

Coat each ball with a teaspoon of chocolate mix, then sprinkle a small amount of salted roasted sunflower seeds on top and return to the fridge to set.

⅓ cup (50g) sunflower seeds
½ cup (80g) mixed seeds (eg. chia, sesame, hemp, pepitas)
½ cup (65g) almonds
4 Medjool dates, pitted
¼ cup (15g) shredded coconut
2 tbsp coconut oil
2 tbsp almond butter
1 tbsp organic cacao powder
1 tbsp (30g) raw honey
1 tsp vanilla paste
3 drops of food-grade tangerine essential oil
Pinch of salt, for the sunflower seeds

RAW CHOCOLATE DRIZZLE

¼ cup (30g) cacao butter
4 tsp coconut oil
¼ cup (25g) organic cacao powder
3 tsp maple syrup
Pinch of pink salt

Cobbers

Eating Cobbers as a kid is a memory that is burned into my mind – not just because of the intense sweetness but also because of losing dental fillings with them! These are such an easy caramel to make, this time without all that sugar and trips to the dentist.

Line a baking tray with greaseproof paper. To make the caramel centre, place ingredients in a food processor or Thermomix, and blend together to form a caramel consistency, scraping down the sides until it is smooth and combined (**TM** speed 6). Tip out onto baking tray, press it down firmly and evenly, then freeze for 25 minutes. Once set, cut into small squares and return to freezer for a few more minutes.

To make the chocolate coating, use the double boiler method over low heat, and melt the cacao butter and coconut oil together (**TM** heat 50, speed 2, 5 minutes). Add the cacao powder, maple syrup, maca and salt and stir together. Remove from heat.

Push a skewer or toothpick into a square of caramel, dip in the chocolate mixture so it is fully coated. Place back on the baking tray. Repeat with all the squares, then return baking tray to the freezer until set, approximately one hour.

NOTES For a smooth caramel, put a sheet of greaseproof paper on your kitchen bench and the caramel mixture on top. Layer another sheet of paper on top, then use a rolling pin to roll out to desired thickness and size. Trim the edges for an even finish.

CARAMEL CENTRE

2 cups (130g) shredded coconut

16 Medjool dates, pitted

1 tsp vanilla paste

¼ tsp pink salt

5 drops of food-grade lemon essential oil

CHOCOLATE COATING

½ cup (60g) cacao butter

4 tsp coconut oil

¾ cup (75g) organic cacao powder

3 tsp maple syrup

1 tsp maca powder

Pinch of pink salt

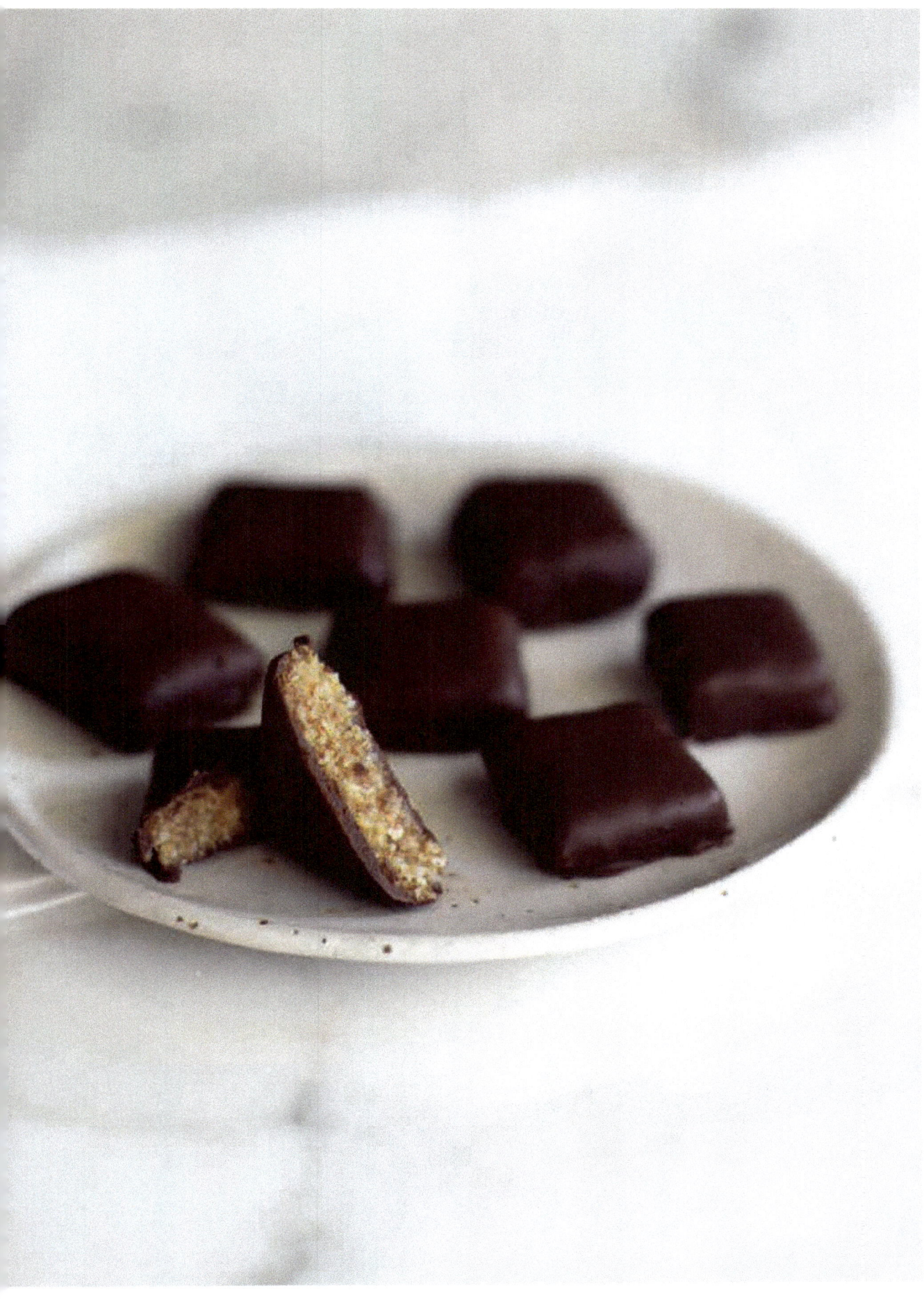

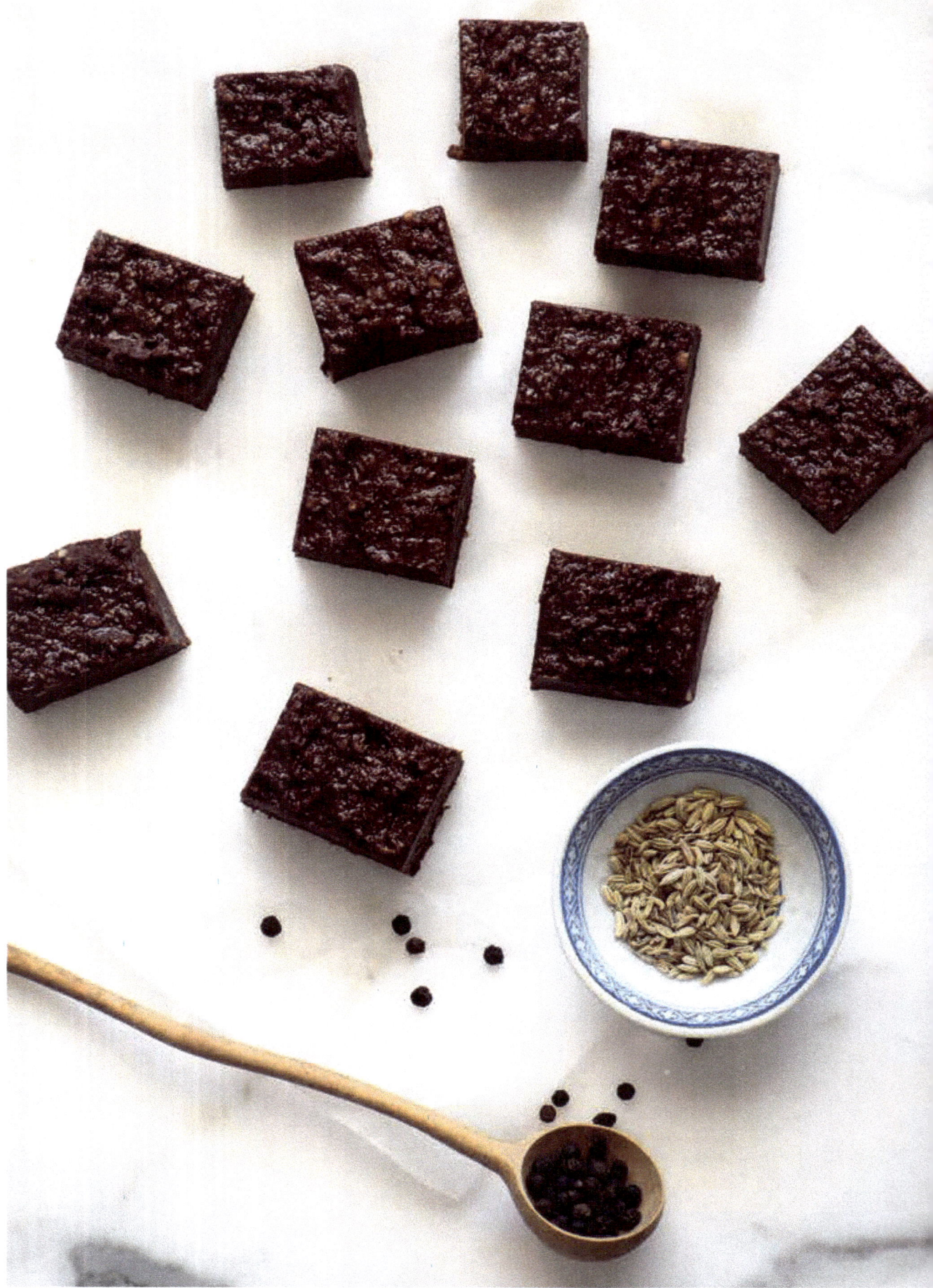

Black Pepper and Fennel Raw Fudge Brownie

The fennel oil used in this recipe brings such a delightful licorice-aniseed touch to the fudge, it really makes it quite grown up and surprising. Fennel is also amazingly supportive to your digestive system and for lactating mothers.

Line a baking tray with greaseproof paper. Add all ingredients a food processor or Thermomix and blend well (**TM** speed 10, 90 seconds), scraping down sides as needed. Once totally combined, tip onto your tray, press down evenly and firmly, and refrigerate until set, approximately one hour.

2 cups (260g) almonds
½ cup (90g) coconut oil
¾ cup (225g) honey
1 cup (100g) organic cacao powder
1 tsp vanilla paste
½ tsp pink salt
1 tbsp maca powder
5 drops food-grade black pepper essential oil
4 drops food-grade fennel essential oil

Florentine

Florentine used to be a weakness for me, but with this version full of healthy fats in the nuts and coconut, I feel totally content and satiated. And there's no sugar crash to deal with!

Line a baking tray with greaseproof paper. Using the double boiler method over low heat, stir together cacao butter, coconut oil and maple syrup until melted (**TM** heat 50, speed 2, 5 minutes), then add all other ingredients and mix well (**TM** reverse speed 2). You want this to be a chunky texture. Spread out onto lined tray and refrigerate for approximately one hour or until set. Cut into squares or slices (as pictured) to serve.

- 1/3 cup (40g) cacao butter
- 1/3 cup (60g) coconut oil
- 3 tbsp (60g) maple syrup
- 2 cups (260g) mixed nuts, roughly chopped
- 1 cup (65g) shredded coconut
- 1/2 cup (60g) goji berries
- 1/2 cup (65g) pepitas
- 1/4 cup (25g) organic cacao powder
- 1/4 cup (35g) dried cranberries
- 1/4 cup (40g) chia seeds
- 1 tsp vanilla paste
- 1 tsp maca powder
- 2 drops food-grade cinnamon essential oil
- 2 drops food-grade cardamom essential oil

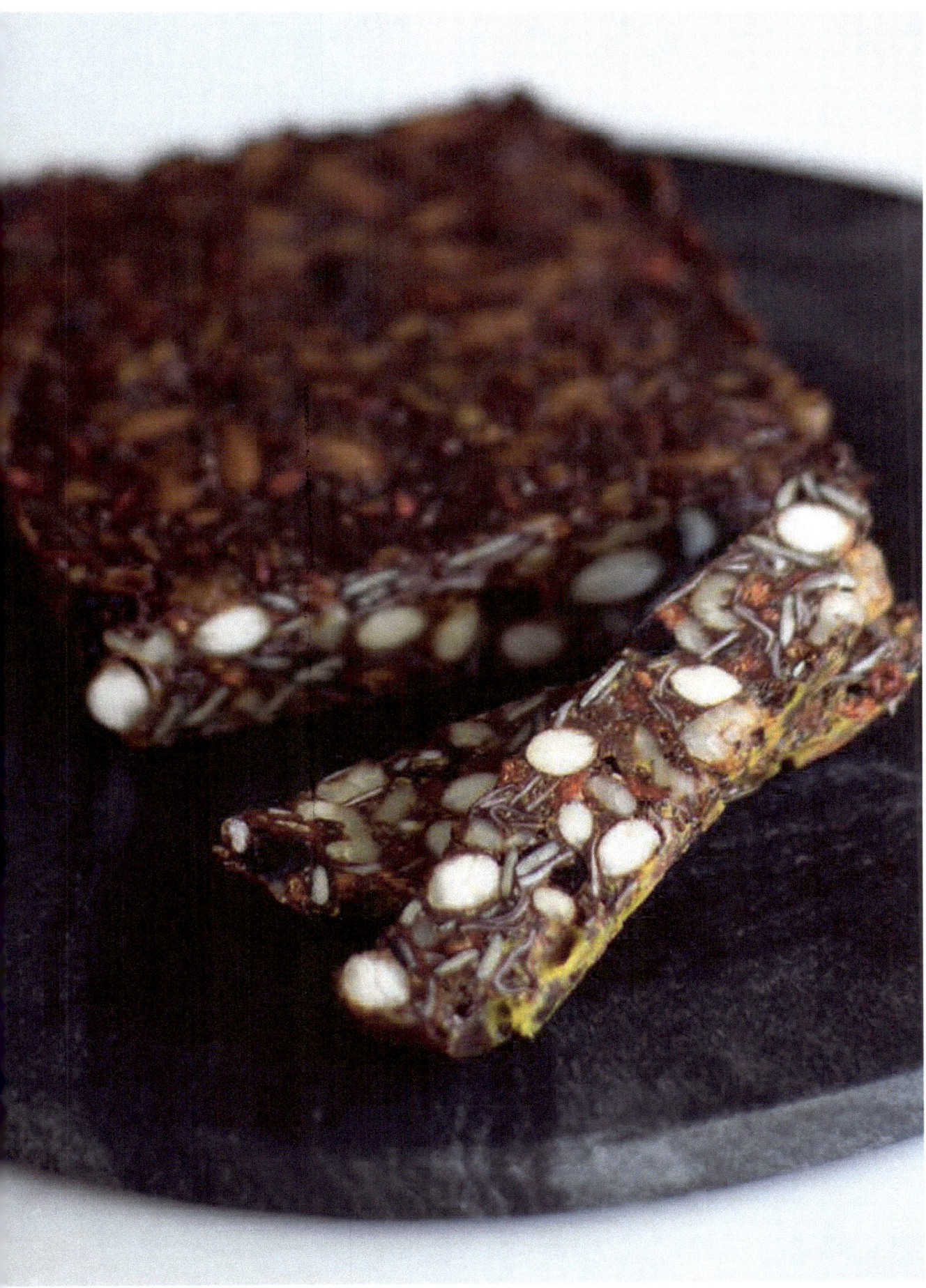

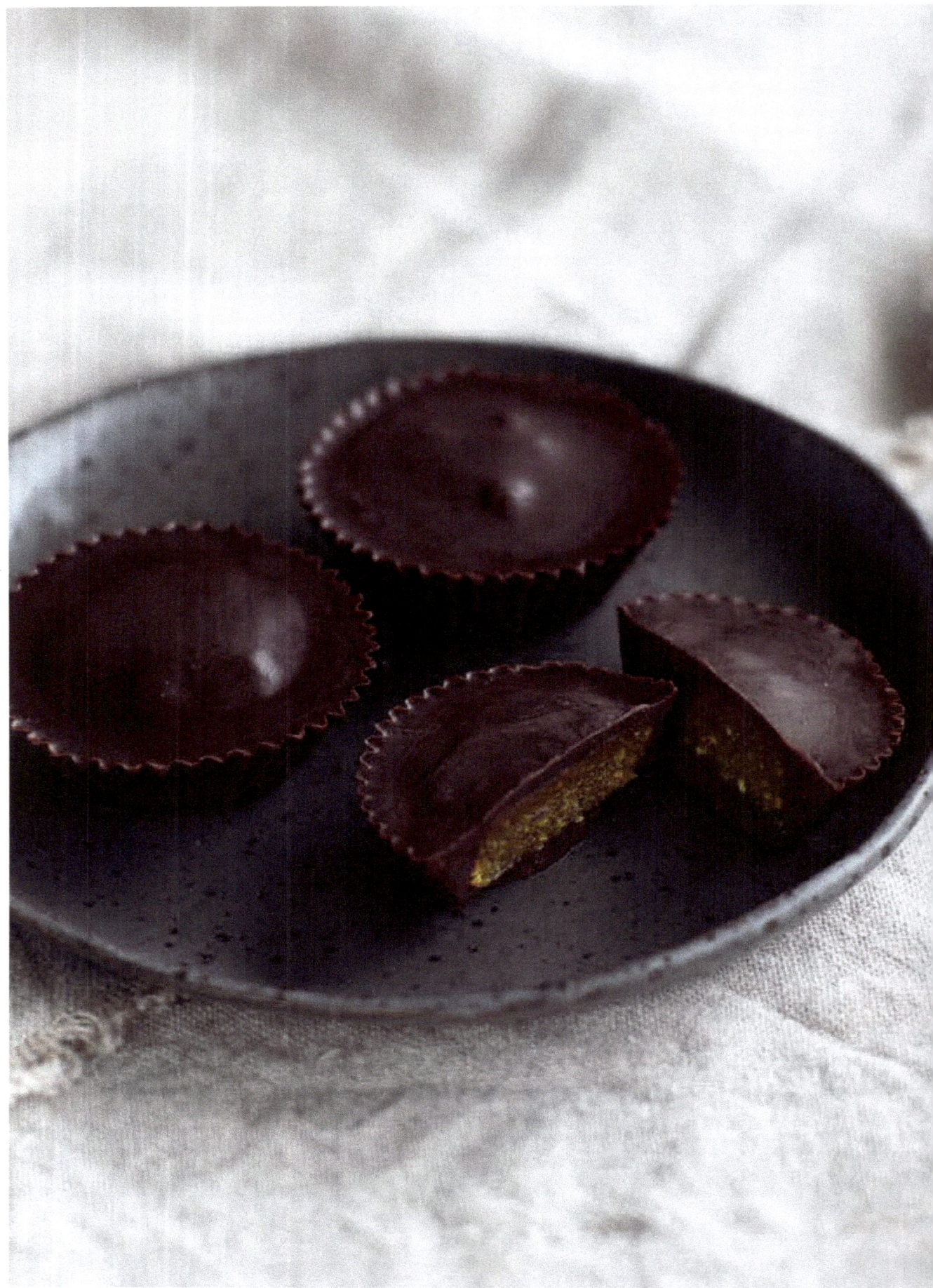

Pistachio Tahini Cups

I love creating surprises inside raw chocolates. Here, one bite delivers a "mouthgasmic" experience – the deluxe intensity of pistachios combined with cinnamon, tahini and golden syrup is unrivalled!

Set around 30 paper patty pans on a flat metal baking tray. Make chocolate by melting cacao butter with coconut oil in a double boiler over low heat, then add cinnamon, salt and maple syrup and stir to combine. Set aside 100ml of the chocolate mixture in a cup with a hot water moat, then divide remaining chocolate mixture between the patty pans (around one teaspoon per patty pan).

Chop pistachio nuts, almond butter, tahini, golden syrup, vanilla, water and coconut oil (**TM** speed 7, scrape down, repeat until you reach a smooth consistency). Place filling into cups. Using the chocolate mixture you have set aside, spoon some over the filling of each cup to create a seal. Refrigerate for one hour or until set.

CHOCOLATE
- 1 cup (120g) cacao butter
- ¼ cup (45g) coconut oil
- 1 cup (100g) organic cacao powder
- ¼ cup maple syrup
- Pinch of pink salt
- 1 tsp maca powder
- 3 drops food-grade cinnamon essential oil

FILLING
- 1 cup (130g) pistachio nuts
- ¼ cup (85g) almond butter
- ¼ cup (70g) tahini
- 3 tbsp golden syrup
- 2-3 tbsp coconut water
- 1 tsp vanilla paste

Puffed Grain Cacao Superfood Bars

This is a variation on a muesli bar using puffed rice, camu camu powder and buckinis. Camu camu delivers a high concentration of vitamin C, plus several phytonutrients and amino acids. Along with the superfoods and citrus oils, it's refreshing and super healthy at the same time. This one is also nut-free so it's school-friendly and incredibly nutrient-dense.

Line a baking tray with greaseproof paper. Using the double boiler method over low heat, melt the coconut oil with the essential oils (**TM** heat 50, reverse speed 3, until melted). Then add all other ingredients in and mix together well (**TM** reverse speed 3, 45 seconds).

Press evenly into baking tray, refrigerate for one hour or until set, then cut into squares.

TIP Add essential oils into the coconut oil to allow even distribution.

½ cup (90g) of coconut oil
5 drops food-grade lemon essential oil
5 drops food-grade lime essential oil
5 drops food-grade wild orange essential oil
3 cups puffed rice (or a mix of puffed grains, eg millet, quinoa, amaranth, brown rice, buckwheat, oats)
½ cup (80g) of buckinis
2 cups (130g) shredded coconut
¼ cup (40g) chia seeds
¼ cup (25g) organic cacao powder
½ cup (140g) maple syrup
¼ cup (30g) cacao nibs
2 tbsp hemp seeds
1 tsp vanilla paste
1 tsp camu camu
Pinch of pink salt

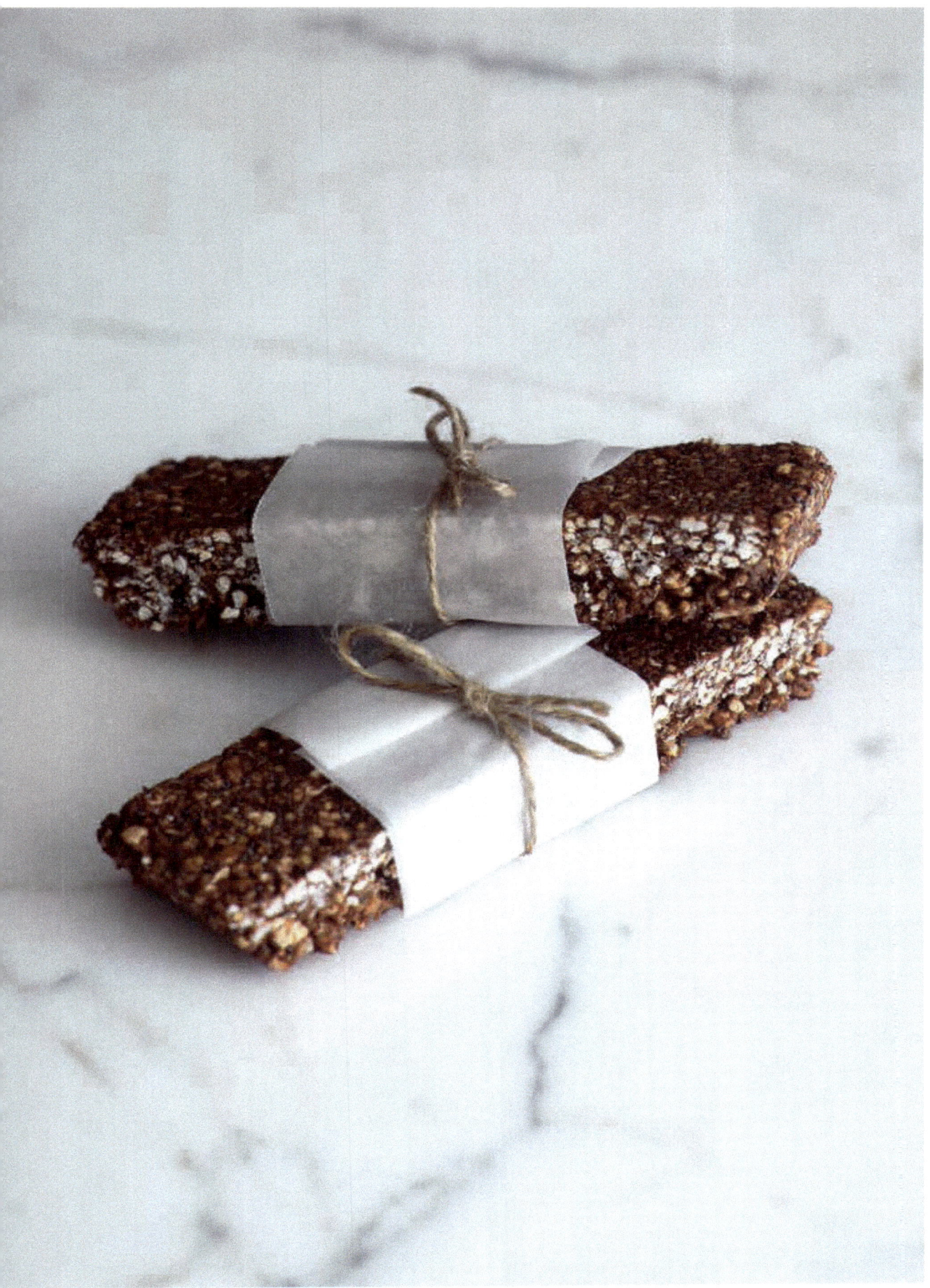

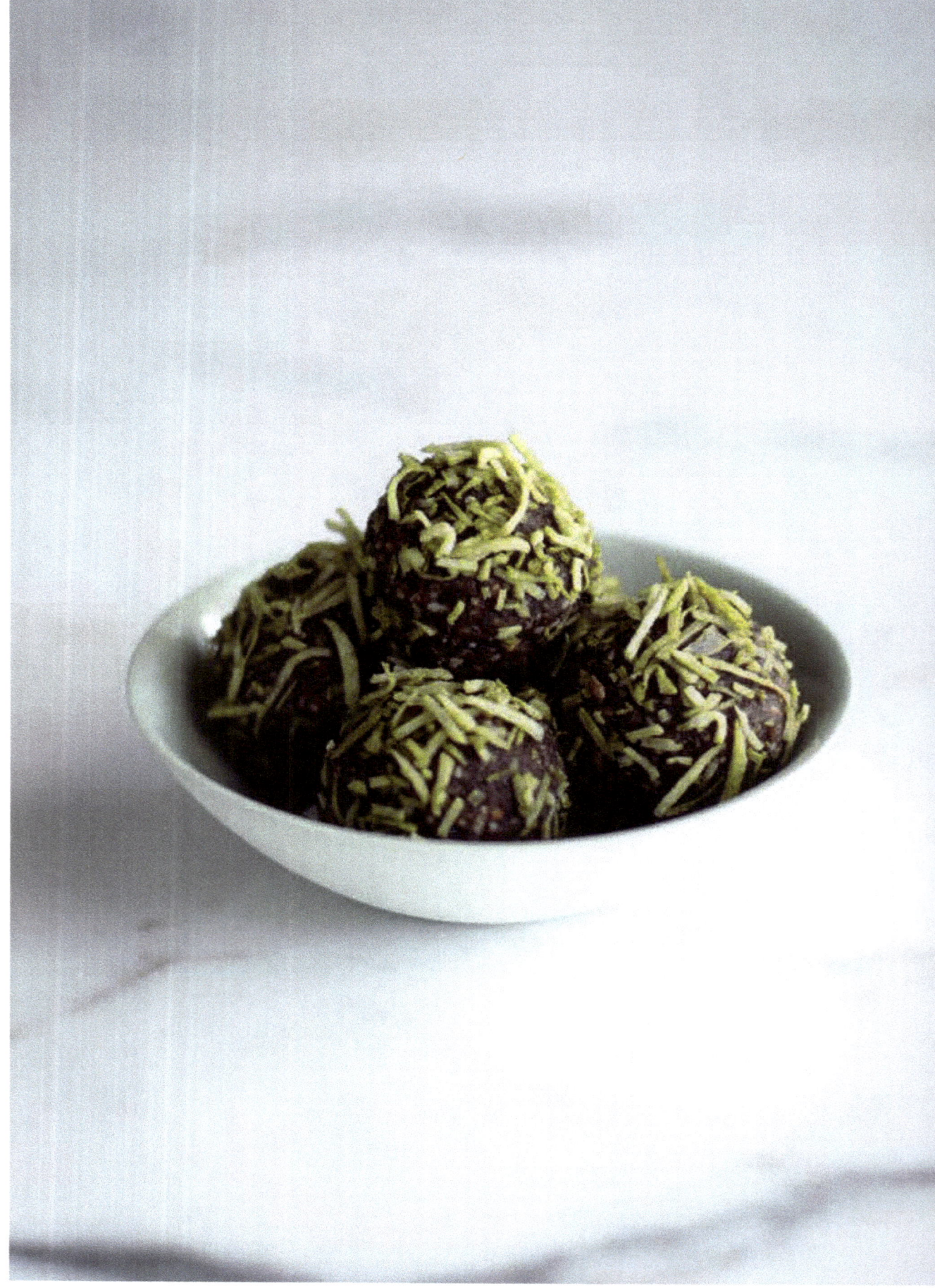

Hemp and Matcha Cardamom Nut Balls

These bliss balls are bursting with goodness – the seeds, hemp protein and nuts deliver good fats and protein, while matcha powder adds quality antioxidants as well as metabolism-boosting properties.

Place all ingredients except matcha powder and extra coconut in a food processor or Thermomix and blend well (**TM** speed 6, scrape down). In a small bowl, combine the matcha powder and rolling coconut.

Roll into small balls, then roll in shredded coconut and matcha powder mix.

Refrigerate until set, approximately one hour.

TIP If the mixture is a little dry after blending, add in more dates or another tablespoon of coconut oil.

½ cup (70g) mixed seeds (eg black sesame, sunflower, pepitas)

½ cup (65g) almonds

⅓ cup (20g) shredded coconut, plus ¼ cup extra for rolling

¼ cup (85g) peanut butter

6 Medjool dates, pitted

4 tbsp (60g) coconut oil

1 tbsp hemp protein

1 tbsp organic cacao powder

½ tsp vanilla paste

3 drops food-grade cardamom essential oil

4 drops food-grade wild orange essential oil

Pinch of pink salt

½ tsp matcha powder

Almond Chocolate with Spiced Pistachio Crackle

The delicate mix of spices used in the crackle here reminds me of an Indian chai – warm, comforting and luxurious. I've also added in some amazing maqui berry powder to bump up the antioxidant healing quota, while the bright green of the pistachios set against the dark brown cacao makes this a feast for the senses.

To make the crackle: Line a baking tray with greaseproof paper. In a bowl, add essential oils to the maple syrup. In a small frypan, toast pistachios over medium heat until lightly browned. Add the maple syrup mix and stir well, until the nuts begin to caramelize. Spread nut mixture on to tray to cool.

To make the chocolate: Line a second baking tray with greaseproof paper. To make the chocolate, chop almonds (**TM** speed 7, 8 seconds) put aside, then in a double boiler over low heat, melt coconut oil and cacao butter (**TM** heat 50, speed 2, 5 minutes), then add remaining ingredients, including the chopped almonds, mixing well (**TM** speed 3, 60 seconds). Pour out on to baking tray, spread evenly.

Once the crackle has cooled, chop into pieces, and sprinkle over the chocolate and refrigerate until set, approx 45 minutes to one hour.

TIP If the crackle hasn't cooled enough and you don't want to wait, you can spoon the warm crackle onto surface of chocolate and spread evenly.

CRACKLE

3 tbsp maple syrup

2 drops food-grade cardamom essential oil

2 drops food-grade cinnamon essential oil

½ cup (65g) pistachios

Pinch of pink salt

CHOCOLATE

2 cups (260g) activated almonds

¼ cup (45g) coconut oil

½ cup (60g) cacao butter

½ cup (50g) organic cacao powder

3 tbsp (45g) maple syrup

2 tbsp hemp seeds

1 tsp vanilla paste

½ tsp maqui powder

¼ tsp pink salt

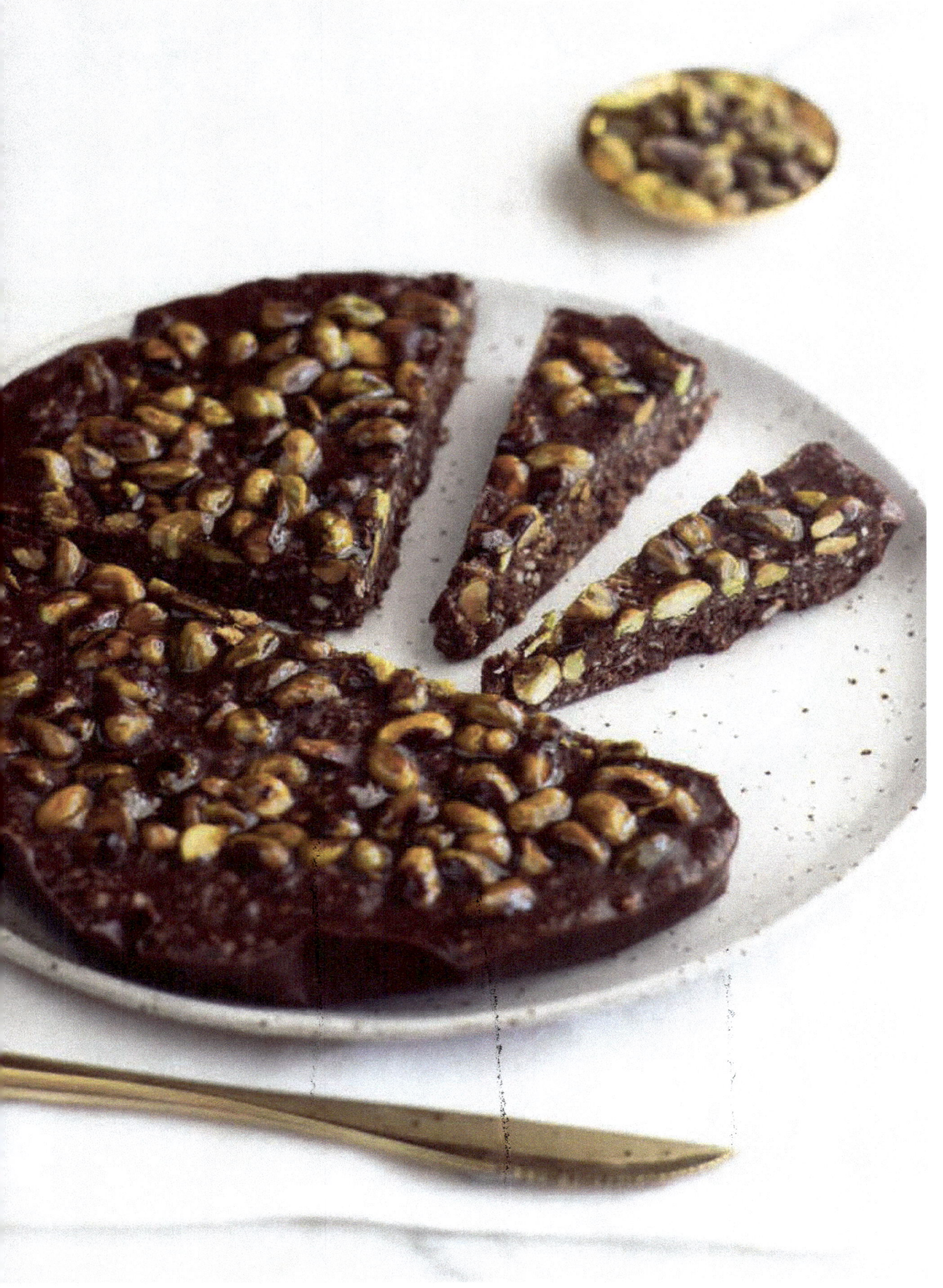

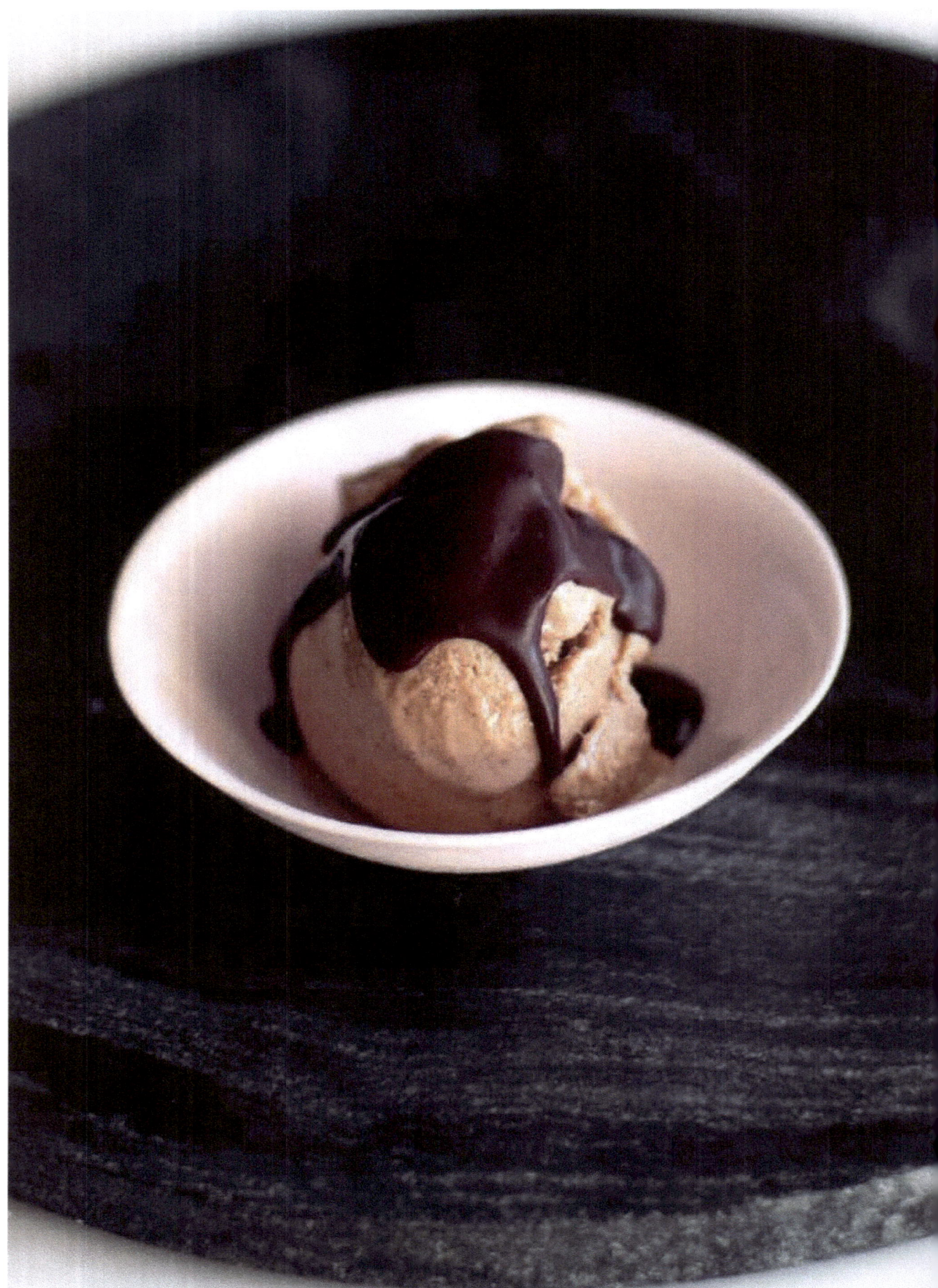

Raw Banana Peanut Butter Ice Cream

Frozen bananas make a creamy, smooth, dairy-free ice cream base which you can layer a variety of flavours over. Get creative and see what you can discover.

Place all ingredients in a blender or Thermomix. Whizz up to a smooth consistency – you will need to scrape down the sides and keep blending until the bananas come together (**TM** speed 10, 90 seconds).

Can be served with nuts, fruit or "nice magic" – just whip up a basic chocolate mixture (see page 28) with melted coconut oil, cacao butter, cacao powder and maple syrup which will set on the ice cream.

TIP Chop up bananas before freezing them to make them easier to blend. This ice cream must be eaten once it has been made, as it will re-freeze into a hard mass. Good excuse to eat all of it!

4 frozen bananas, chopped
2 heaped tbsp peanut butter
100g coconut cream
1 tbsp organic cacao powder
1 tbsp maple syrup
½ tsp pink salt
½ tsp vanilla paste
1-2 drops of your choice of food-grade essential oils (eg cardamom, cinnamon, orange)

Tangerine Mousse

I think mousse deserves a comeback as a wonderful dessert to serve. This version is just as decadent, but without the heaviness of cream and introducing the bright, light notes of tangerine.

Approximately half an hour before starting the recipe, place the tin of coconut cream in the freezer.

Scrape out into a glass or metal bowl the cream part of the tin (don't shake it so the fat content stays on the top), and then set aside the extra watery milk left in the tin. With an electric hand beater, start to slowly mix the cream, adding all other ingredients until it thickens. This takes around 2-3 minutes.

Divide into four small bowls and refrigerate for 45 minutes to one hour, then serve with raspberries and/or cacao nibs

400ml tin coconut cream
1 tbsp coconut butter, melted
1 heaped tbsp raw honey (or more depending on sweetness)
4 tbsp organic cacao powder
4 drops food-grade tangerine essential oil
½ tsp vanilla paste
Pinch of pink salt
Fresh raspberries or cacao nibs, to serve

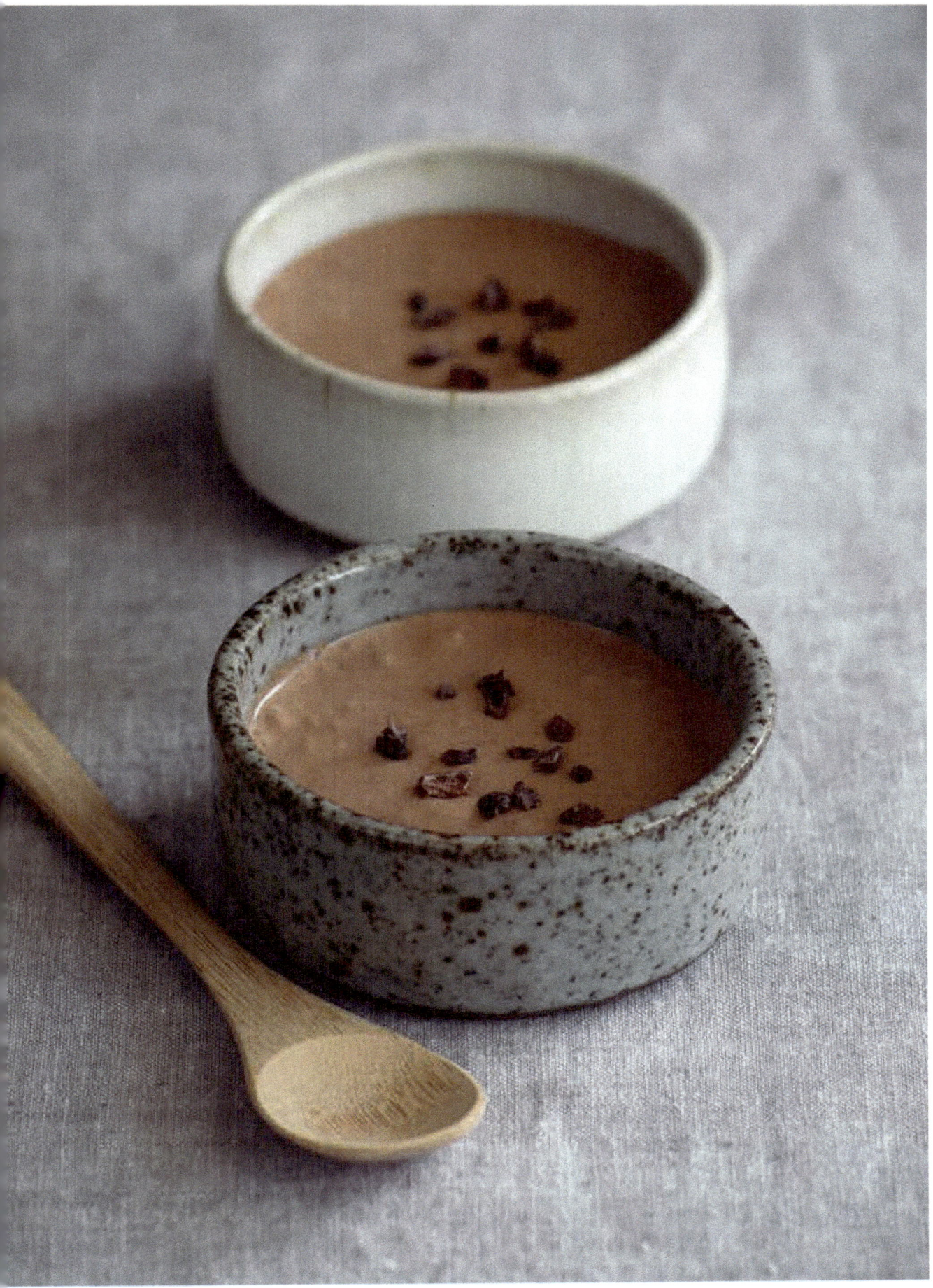

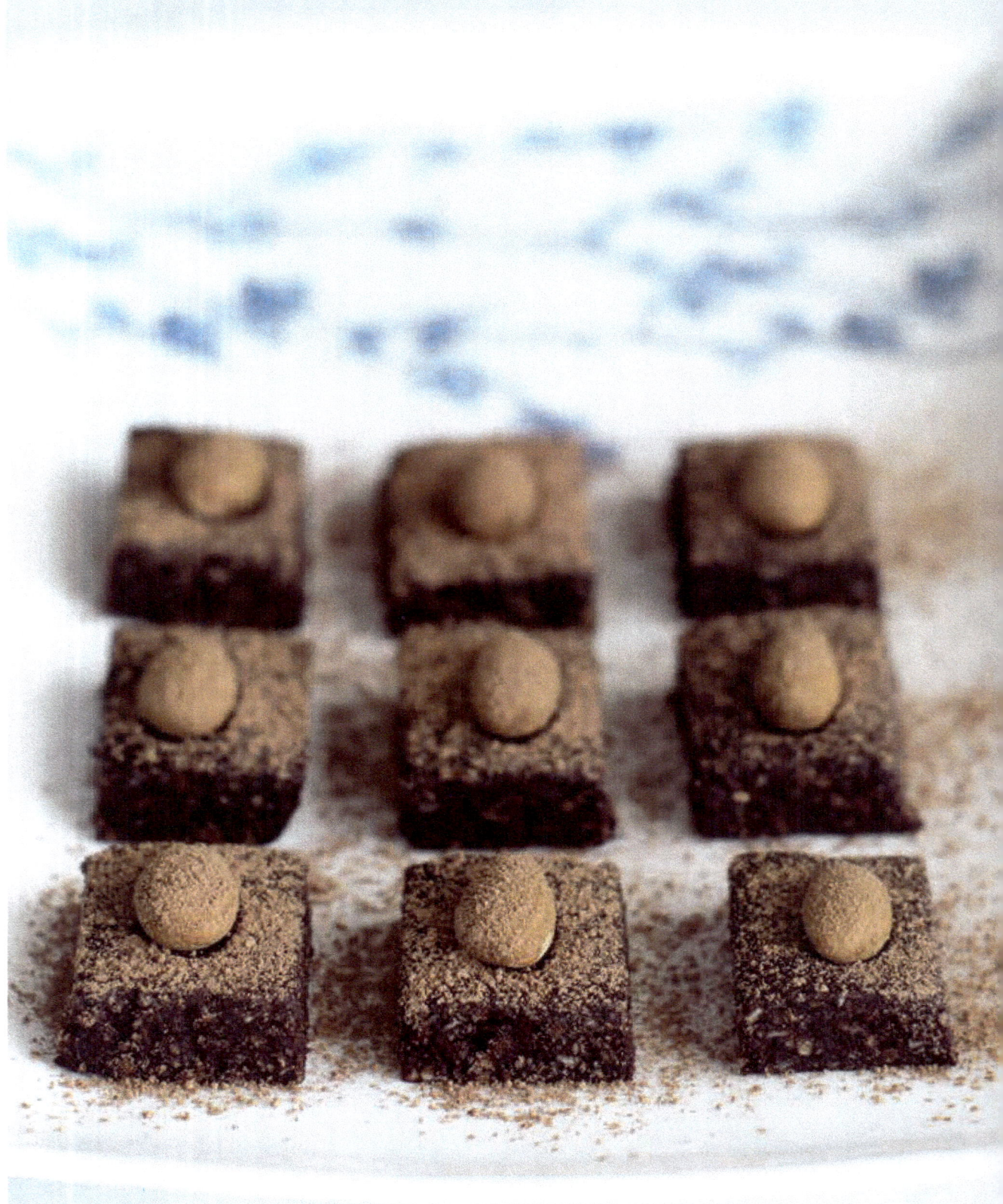

Raw Almond Cacao Fudge

Most of us find a piece of fudge fairly irresistible, so I have created this easy recipe for a fast afternoon treat. "Activating" nuts is the process of soaking and then drying them out – this process increases the nutrient density and also makes them more digestible. You can buy nuts already activated or you can do it easily at home. See page 25 on how to do it.

Line a baking tray with greaseproof paper. In a small saucepan over low heat, melt coconut oil (**TM** 50 degrees, speed 2, 60-90 seconds). Pour melted coconut oil into a food processor and add remaining ingredients. Blend everything together on speed 4 mixing well, scraping down sides (**TM** speed 7, 30 seconds, scrape down sides, repeat). Spread out and press into tray, placing an almond evenly across the surface of fudge (so when it is cut you'll have an almond on each piece), and then refrigerate for approximately one hour, or until set.

TIP Scrunch up some greaseproof paper, rub a little coconut oil on the paper and use it to spread out mixture evenly into the tray. Smooth with the back of a tablespoon.

- 1 cup (180g) coconut oil
- 2 cups (260g) activated almonds, plus some extra for decoration
- 1 cup (100g) organic cacao powder
- ½ cup (150g) honey
- ½ tsp pink salt
- 1 tsp vanilla
- 1 tsp maca powder
- 3 drops food-grade cinnamon essential oil

Spiced Cacao Chai Balls with a Crunch

These balls are exotic, warming, satisfying and completely grounding. I use a Protective Blend of wild orange, eucalyptus, rosemary, clove and cinnamon essential oils plus other oils including cardamom, ginger and fennel – it's an amazing immune system booster.

In a food processor or Thermomix, chop almonds to a rough texture (**TM** speed 4, 10 seconds), then add dates, coconut oil, cacao, seeds, vanilla, salt and essential oils. Mix again until combined (**TM** speed 6, 60 seconds). Add in nibs and mix through – do not chop as you want these whole for crunch (**TM** reverse speed 3, 10 seconds). Roll into balls and refrigerate for one hour or until set.

TIP To get the balls to roll easily without sticking, I have found it useful to wear disposable gloves with just a touch of coconut oil rubbed together.

1 cup (130g) activated almonds
12 Medjool dates, pitted
3 tbsp (45g) coconut oil
3 tbsp (20g) organic cacao powder
2 tbsp hemp seeds
1 tbsp chia seeds
1 tsp vanilla paste
1 tsp maqui powder
4 drops food-grade cardamom essential oil
4 drops food-grade ginger essential oil
4 drops food-grade Protective Blend essential oil
4 drops food-grade fennel essential oil
4 drops food-grade black pepper essential oil
Big pinch of pink salt
¼ cup (30g) cacao nibs

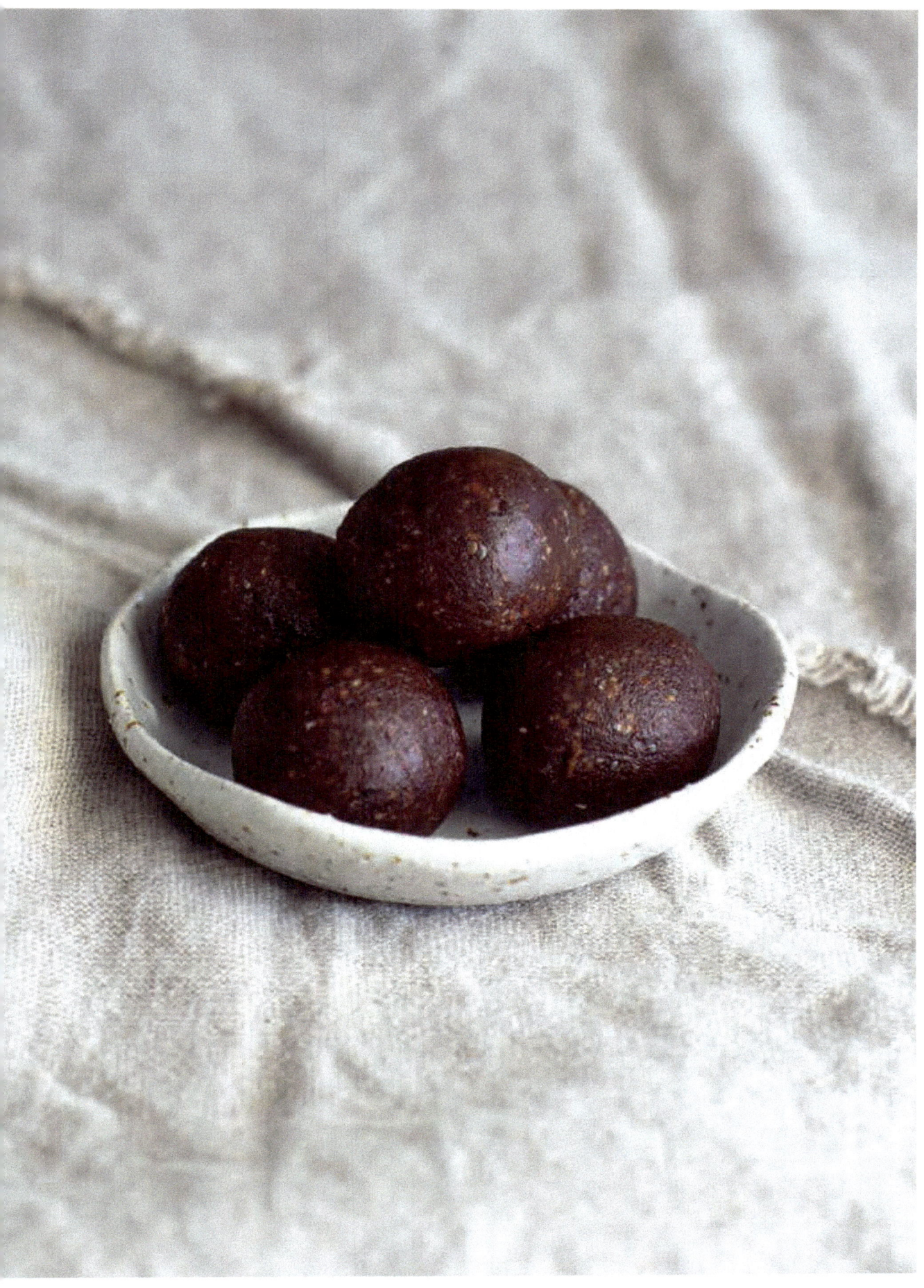

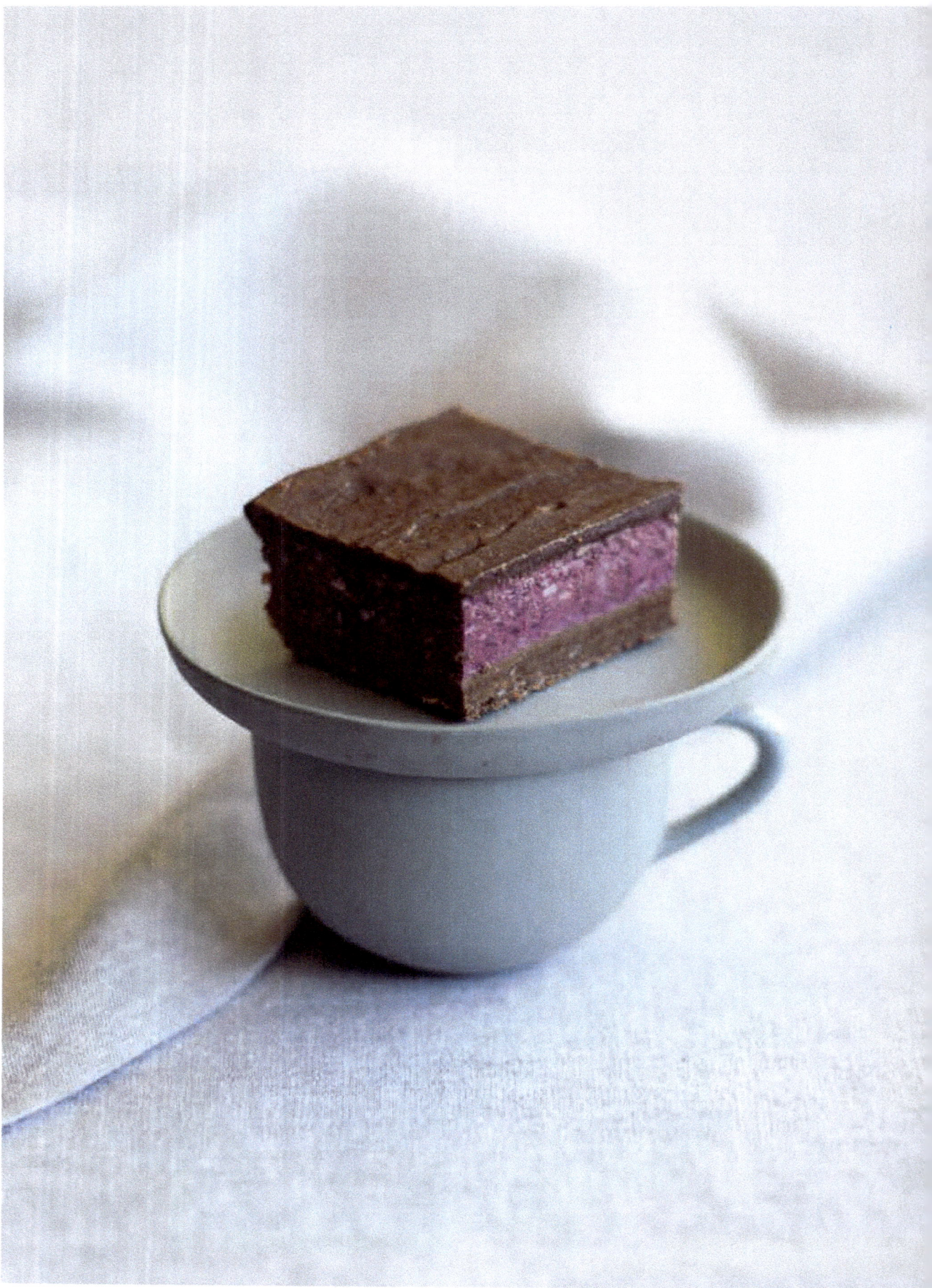

Raw Chocolate Raspberry Slice

It might look like a lot of components to pull together for this slice, but just think of it as making three easy things, and then combining them. You'll be surprised at how quickly you are sitting down with a cup of tea and enjoying this impressive reward.

To make the base: Line a square tray with greaseproof paper. In a food processor or Thermomix, chop the almonds, cacao and coconut (**TM** speed 7, scrape down, repeat until well combined). Add melted coconut oil, dates, essential oil and chop again (**TM** speed 3, 1-2 minutes). Scrape down and repeat as needed until everything is well combined. Press this mixture into the tray and put in the freezer to chill while you make the next layer.

To make the raspberry layer: Put all ingredients in a food processor or Thermomix, and blend until it comes together (**TM** speed 5, 1-2 minutes, scrape down sides). You can add extra maple syrup if desired. Pour this over the top of the base layer and return to the freezer to set before topping with the chocolate layer.

To make the chocolate layer: In a double boiler over low heat, melt coconut oil before whisking in other ingredients (**TM** melt coconut oil, 37 degrees, speed 2, 30 seconds; then add all other ingredients mixing well, speed 3, 60 seconds).

Pour this layer over the raspberry layer and place it back in the freezer to set. Work quickly to avoid the chocolate layer setting too fast due to the cold raspberry layer.

Remove from the freezer when firm (approximately two hours), and slice with a serrated knife into desired sizes.

Store in the freezer, bring to room temperature about 15 minutes before serving.

BASE LAYER
- 1 cup (130g) almonds
- 1/3 cup (35g) organic cacao powder
- 1/3 cup (20g) shredded coconut
- 4 tbsp (60g) coconut oil, melted
- 6 Medjool dates, pitted and soaked for 2 hours
- 2 tbsp maple syrup
- 6 drops food-grade wild orange essential oil

RASPBERRY LAYER
- 2 cups (240g) fresh or frozen raspberries or mixed berries
- 1/3 cup (30g) shredded coconut
- 1/3 cup (90g) pure maple syrup
- 1 tbsp chia seeds
- 1 cup (130g) raw cashews, soaked overnight, drained

TOP LAYER
- 1/3 cup (60g) coconut oil
- 1/3 cup (35g) organic cacao powder
- 1/4 cup (70g) pure maple syrup
- 3 tbsp cacao nibs
- Pinch of pink salt
- 10 drops food-grade lime essential oil

Chia Cardamom Orange Pudding

Chia seeds are little dynamos – a great source of protein, packed with omega-3 fatty acids, rich in antioxidants, and they also provide fibre, iron and calcium. Because they don't have a dominant flavour, they can morph into a range of desserts effortlessly.

Place all ingredients into a glass bowl and whisk until combined. Allow to sit for 5 minutes, then whisk again. Repeat this 2 or 3 times. Place in the fridge to set for approximately 45 minutes to one hour. Spoon out into small serving bowls and garnish with chopped nuts, coconut flakes or fresh berries.

TIP For a different consistency, you can blitz everything up for a smoother feel and then place straight in the fridge. I personally like the texture leaving the chia seeds whole as it has somewhat of a nostalgic tapioca pudding feel.

1 ½ cups (375g) almond or coconut milk
⅓ cup (50g) chia seeds
¼ cup (25g) organic cacao powder
3 tbsp (50g) maple syrup
1 tsp vanilla paste
1 tsp acai powder
1 drop food-grade cardamom essential oil
2 drops food-grade wild orange essential oil
Pinch of pink salt
Chopped mixed nuts, coconut flakes or fresh berries, to serve

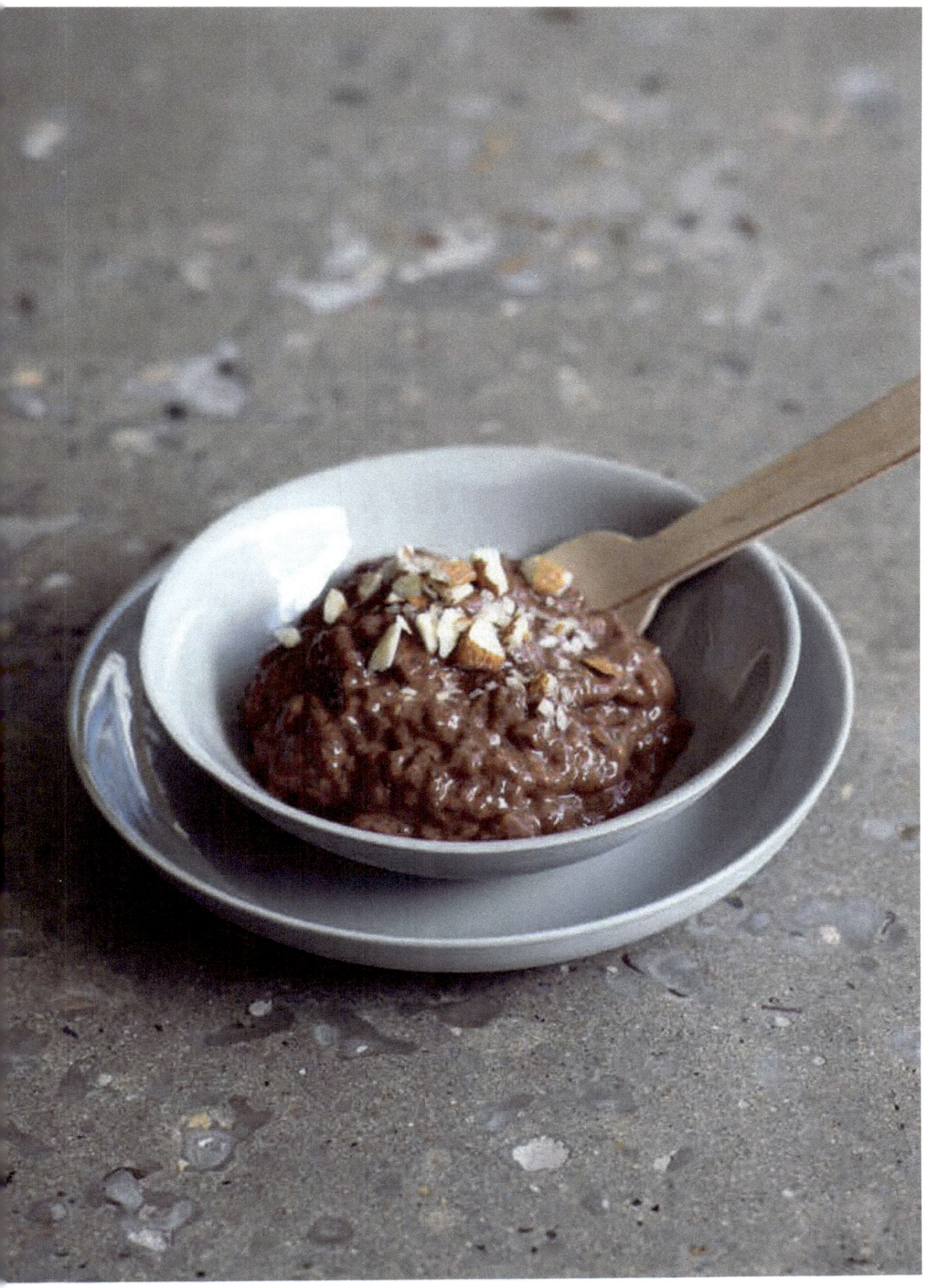

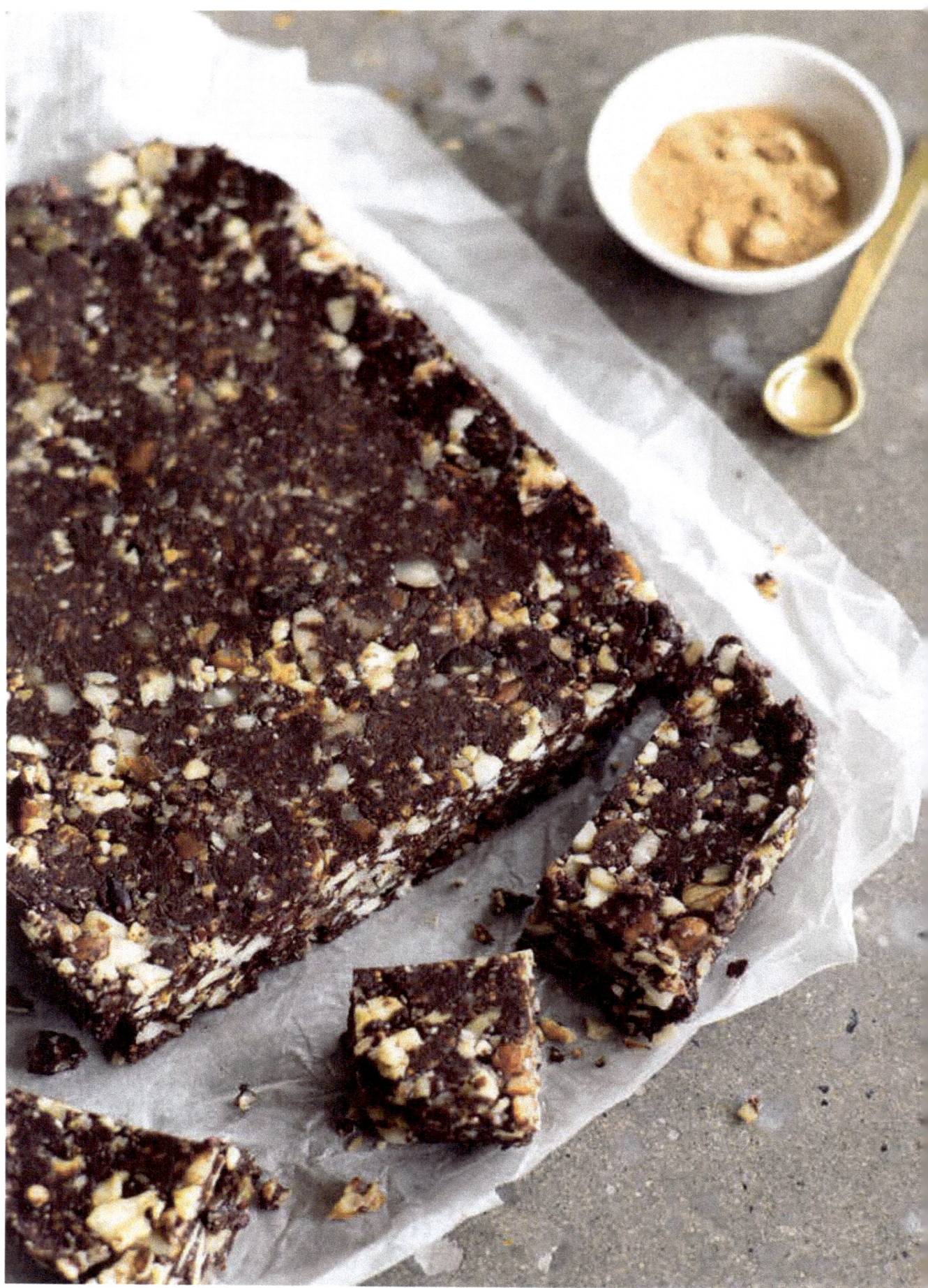

Immunity Boosting Raw Cacao Cake Slab

The ingredients in this cake slab are highly nutritious, health-boosting and rich with antioxidants. Copaiba essential oil is distilled from a South American tree resin. Copaiba has been used by South American shamans and people to support overall mind-body health and healing, so when combined with other powerful oils and camu camu powder's amino acids and vitamin C, this slab really packs a punch!

Line a baking tray with greaseproof paper. In a small saucepan over low heat, melt coconut oil (**TM** 50 degrees, speed 2, 30 seconds), then chop all other ingredients on a low speed, mixing well (**TM** speed 3, 25 seconds). Press down evenly and firmly into lined tray. Refrigerate for one hour or until set. Serve whole on a wooden board for an impressive dessert. This can also be cut into slices and kept small for individual treats.

TIP For more on the Protective Blend, see page 68.

¼ cup (45g) coconut oil
2 cups (260g) mixed nuts
½ cup (50g) organic cacao powder
⅓ cup (45g) white mulberries
⅓ cup (20g) shredded coconut
¼ cup (40g) activated buckinis
¼ cup (30g) pepitas
4 tbsp (45g) maple syrup
3 tbsp amaranth flakes
2 tbsp chia seeds
2 tbsp hemp seeds
1 tsp maca powder
1 tsp camu camu
½ tsp spirulina powder
¼ tsp pink salt
2 tbsp cacao nibs
8 drops food-grade Protective Blend essential oil
5 drops food-grade black pepper essential oil
2 drops food-grade copaiba essential oil

Cacao Butter Superfood Balls

This variation of cacao without the addition of cacao powder, adds a new dimension to bliss balls. These balls contain such a dense amount of superfoods that each bite delivers a perfect portion of energy, vitality and happiness! Lucuma is a Peruvian fruit that we can use in dried powder form, and brings a host of benefits to the party such as lots of antioxidants, vitamins and minerals such as calcium, zinc and iron.

In a double boiler over low heat (**TM** heat 50, speed 2, 5 minutes) melt coconut oil and cacao butter together, then transfer this to a food processor (**TM** leave in bowl). Add in all other ingredients, and then blitz until slightly chunky (**TM** speed 5 for 35 seconds). The mixture should not be reduced to a meal consistency.

Shape into balls and refrigerate for one hour or until set.

TIP This mixture is a wetter mix, therefore can't really be rolled, rather shaped, but they will form and set when refrigerated.

Ingredients
¼ cup (30g) cacao butter
2 tbsp coconut oil
1 cup (130g) mixed pecans/Brazil nuts
2 tbsp cranberries
3 dried figs
2 tbsp goji berries
2 tbsp sesame seeds
2 tbsp sunflower seeds
2 tsp chia seeds
1 tbsp hemp seeds
2 tbsp pepitas
1 tsp lucuma powder
1 tbsp honey
2 drops of food-grade spearmint essential oil
Pinch of salt

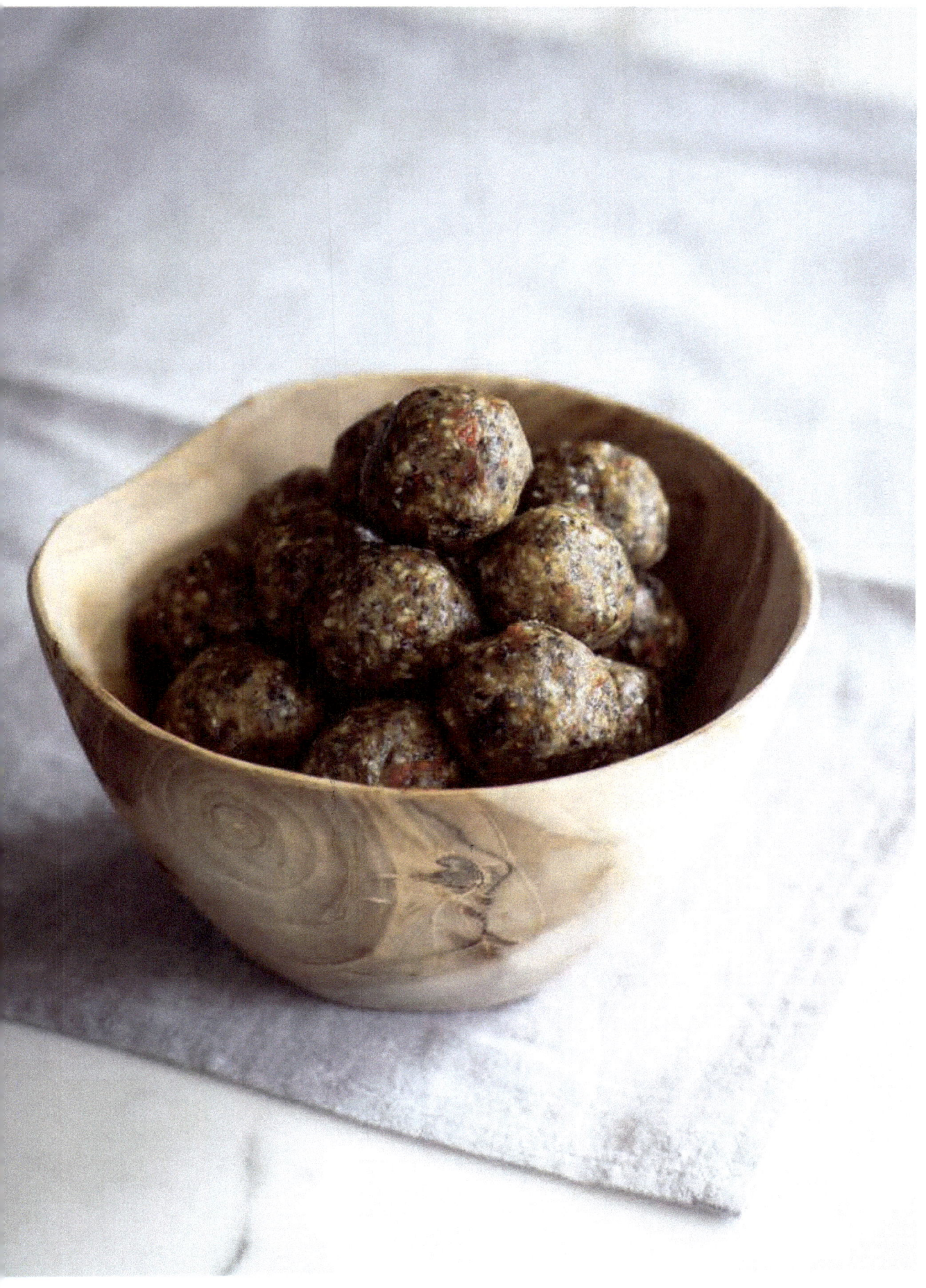

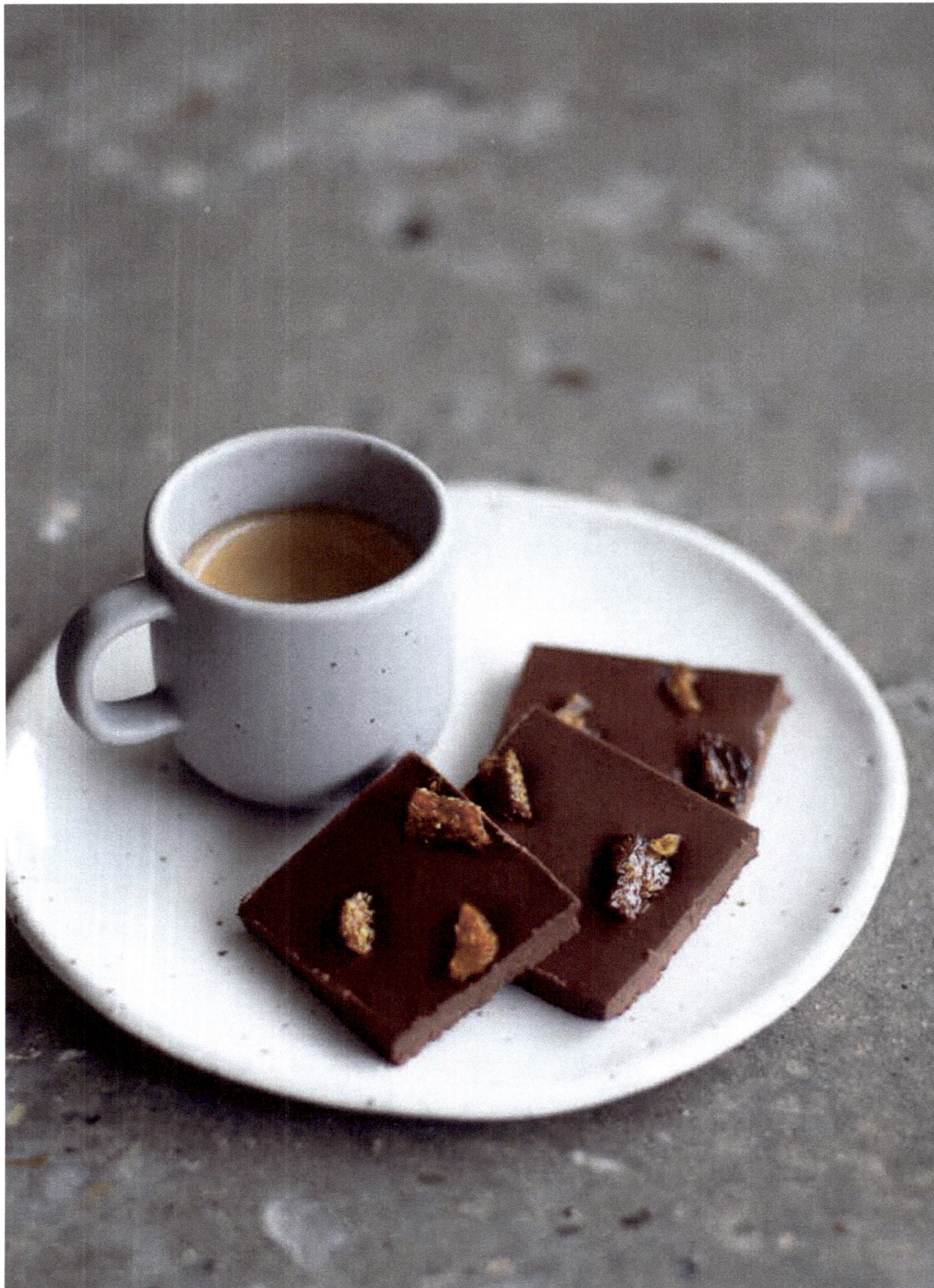

Lemon Myrtle Mylk Chocolate with Inca Berries

This is a nice variation for those who like a lighter chocolate taste. Inca berries are wonderful to have in your pantry as they add so much in the way of nutrition, but also texture, flavour and colour. The berries are high in protein, vitamins A, B and C, and offer a good amount of fibre for a dried fruit. Here, they are a lovely contrast to the smooth velvety coconut chocolate.

Line a baking tray with greaseproof paper or use a silicone mat. In a double boiler over low heat, melt the cacao butter and coconut oil (**TM** heat 50, speed 2, 5 minutes) then add cacao powder, coconut milk, maple syrup, essential oils, salt and mix well (**TM** speed 3).

Pour out the chocolate mixture onto the tray, then place the Inca berries over the surface. Refrigerate for approximately one hour or until set. Cut into squares before serving.

- ½ cup (60g) cacao butter
- 3 tbsp coconut oil
- ½ cup (50g) organic cacao powder
- 100ml coconut milk
- 3 tbsp maple syrup
- 2-3 drops food-grade lemon myrtle essential oil
- Pinch of pink salt
- 2 tbsp Inca berries, chopped

Cardamom Cacao Caramelised Roasted Nut Slab

This is probably one of the most requested recipes to make, as everyone loves roasted nuts, and the honey caramelized taste combined with the flavour of cardamom chocolate, it has everyone drooling for more.

Line a tray with greaseproof paper. In a large frypan over medium heat, dry roast the nuts until slightly toasted. Do not leave them unattended – they can burn quickly. Turn the heat down to low, then slowly add honey bit by bit, stirring through until all nuts are coated and start to bubble and caramelize (just be careful the pan isn't too hot as they will scorch quickly). Pour out nut mix evenly into your tray, rearranging quickly to spread out into an even thickness. When this cools it becomes very sticky and hard to move around.

In a double boiler over low heat or using a Thermomix, melt the cacao butter and coconut oil together (**TM** heat 50, speed 2, 5 minutes), then add in all other ingredients, mixing well for a few minutes. Drizzle chocolate as evenly as possible over the nuts and refrigerate for one hour or until set.

Remove whole slab from tray onto a board and chunk into bits for serving.

Ingredients
4 cups (520g) assorted nuts (your choice, eg macadamia, pistachio, almond, cashew, pecan)
6 tbsp raw honey
1½ cups (180g) cacao butter
⅓ cup (60g) coconut oil
⅓ cup (90g) maple syrup
1½ cups (150g) organic cacao powder
Pinch of pink salt
3-4 drops food-grade cardamom essential oil
1 tsp maca powder

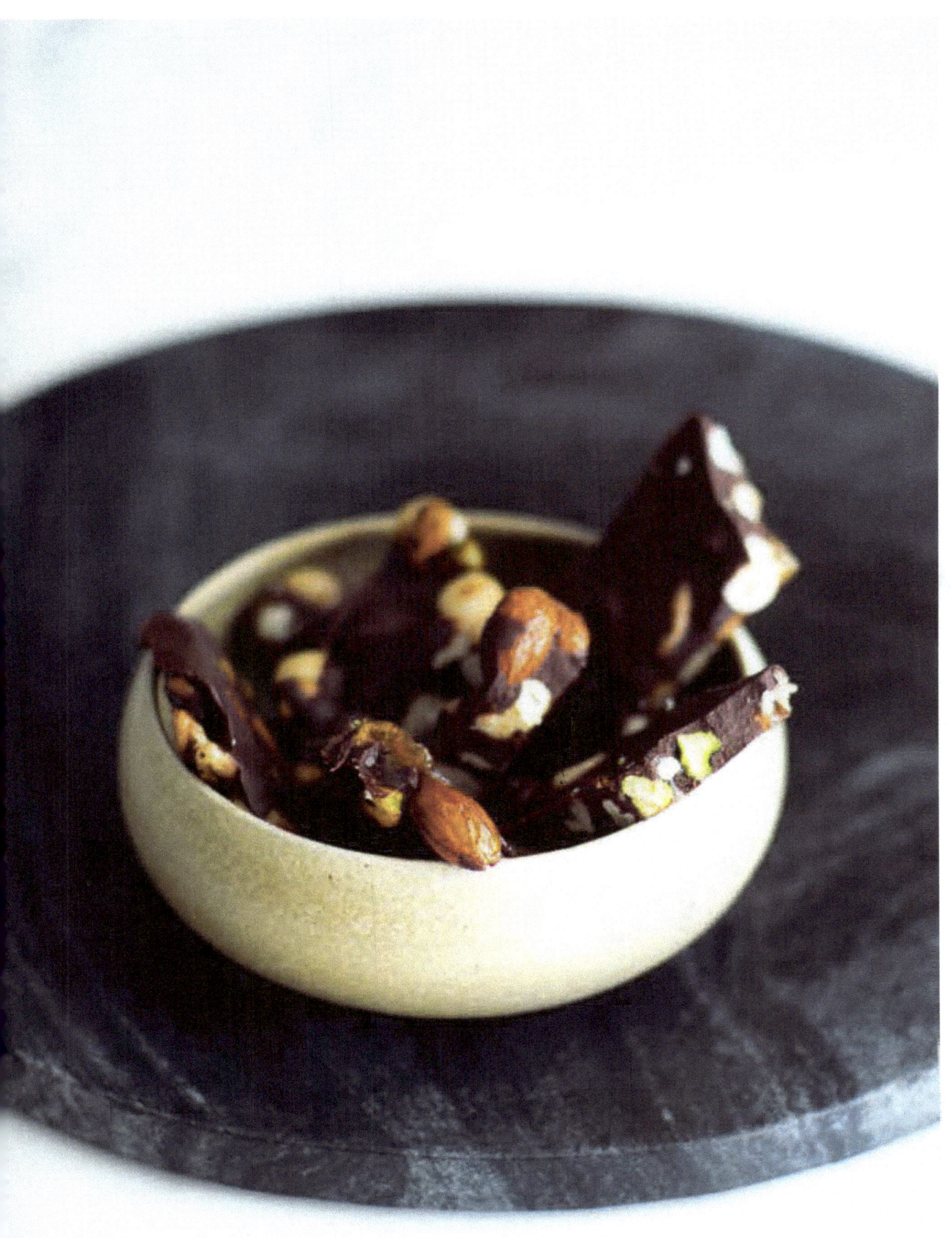

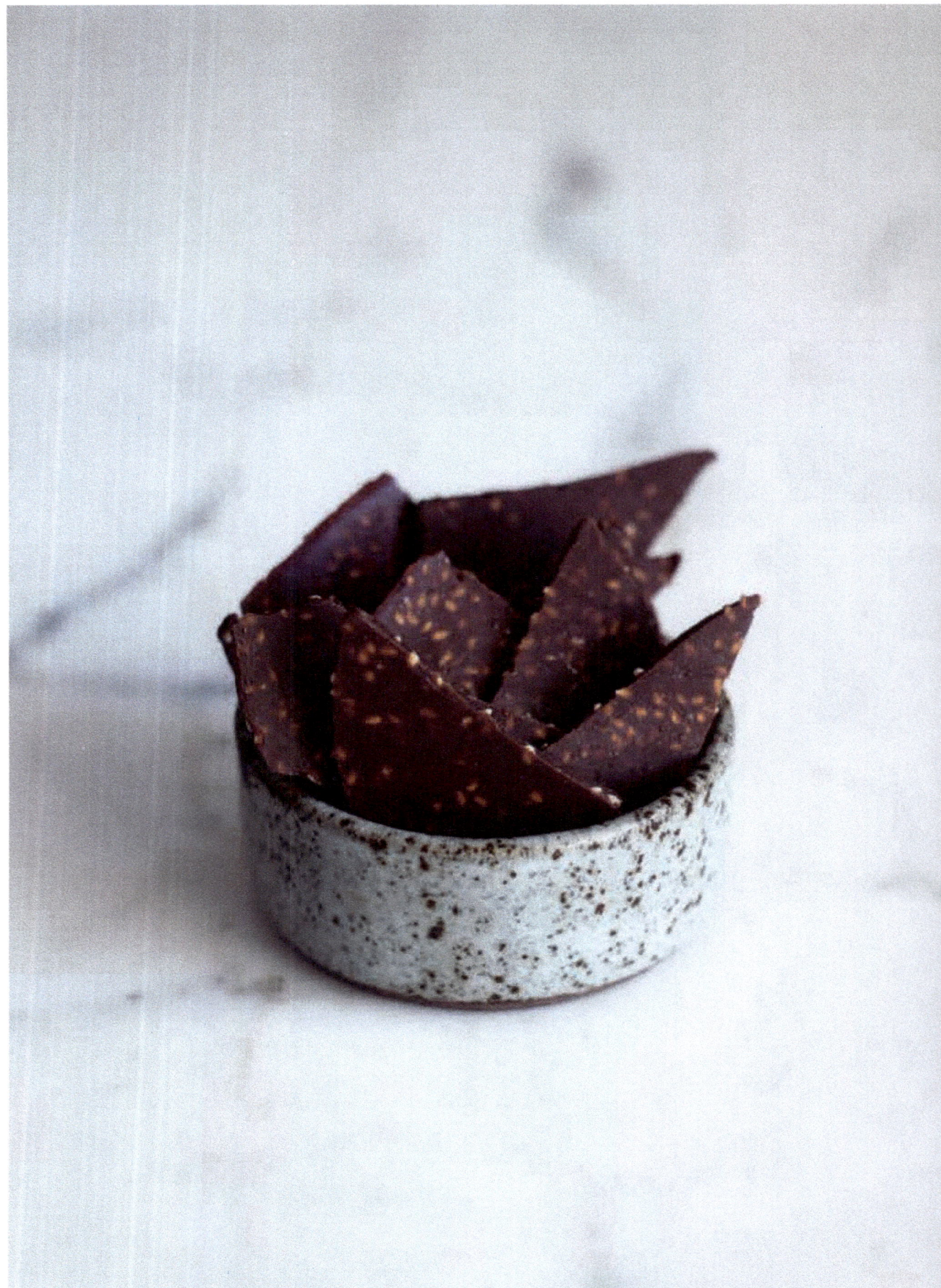

Fennel and Sesame Chocolate

I like to spear shards of this chocolate into ice cream for a quick but impressive dessert. The aniseed flavour of the fennel essential oil and salty contrast makes it pretty sophisticated.

Line a medium to large tray with greaseproof paper. In a double boiler over low heat, stir together cacao butter and coconut oil until they melt (**TM** heat 50, speed 2, 5 minutes). Add all other ingredients and mix well. Pour onto tray, smooth out evenly and refrigerate for approximately 45 minutes to one hour or until set. Crack into pieces before serving.

½ cup (60g) cacao butter

⅓ cup (60g) coconut oil

¼ cup (70g) maple syrup

½ cup (50g) organic cacao powder

½ tsp pink salt

3 drops food-grade fennel essential oil

¼ cup (35g) sesame seeds, lightly toasted

1 tsp maca powder

Matcha Soft Centre Chocolates

I've said it before, but I'll say it again – cashews are the king of versatility. I adore how they lend such a luxurious creaminess to this filling, not to mention a certain degree of satisfaction when eating them, knowing you are eating something so delicious that is actually also good for you. Matcha green tea powder is a powerful addition to these chocolates – it is made from nutrient-dense young green tea leaves, and then stored away from light and air to preserve its wonderful bright green colour.

I usually make this recipe as a chocolate cup in patty pans but it can be easily transformed into a chocolate (as pictured) using moulds. Just follow the steps below but replace patty pans with a hard chocolate mould instead.

Set roughly 20 paper patty pans on a baking tray. For the chocolate, melt cacao butter and coconut oil on low heat in a double boiler (**TM** heat 50, speed 2, 5 minutes), then add in all other ingredients and mix well (**TM** speed 2, 2-3 minutes). Spoon a small amount into the bottom of each patty tin and spin it around to coat up the sides. Brush or spoon some extra chocolate mix up the sides of each patty pan to strengthen the chocolate cup. Refrigerate to set, approximately 10 minutes.

Place all filling ingredients in a food processor or Thermomix, and blend well with a touch of coconut water to make a smooth paste (**TM** speed 8, 1-2 minutes, scrape down sides a few times).

Once the chocolate cups are set, spoon a small amount of cashew filling into the chocolate patty pans, pressing down firmly. Cover with more chocolate to make a lid, then return to the fridge to set for approximately one hour.

CHOCOLATE
- 1 cup (120g) cacao butter
- ¼ cup (45g) coconut oil
- 1 cup (100g) organic cacao powder
- 4 tbsp (80g) maple syrup
- 1 tsp maca powder
- 10 drops food-grade lemon essential oil
- Pinch of pink salt

FILLING
- 1 cup (130g) cashew nuts, soaked overnight in filtered water, then drained
- 2-3 tbsp (40g) almond butter
- 2-3 tbsp (40g) tahini
- 2-3 tbsp (60g) maple syrup
- 1 tsp coconut oil
- ½ tsp matcha powder
- 6 drops food-grade lime essential oil
- 1-2 tbsp coconut water
- Pinch of pink salt

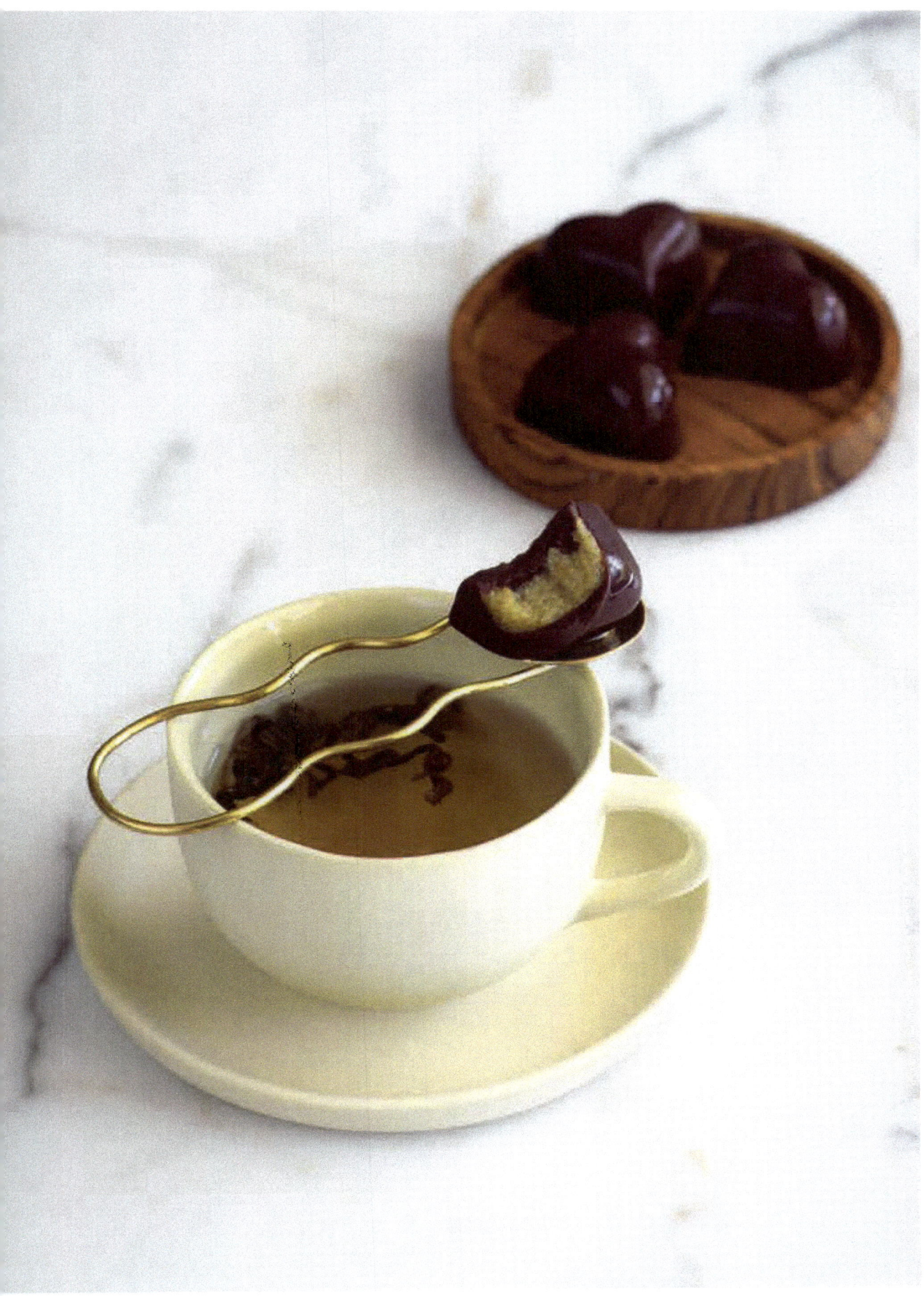

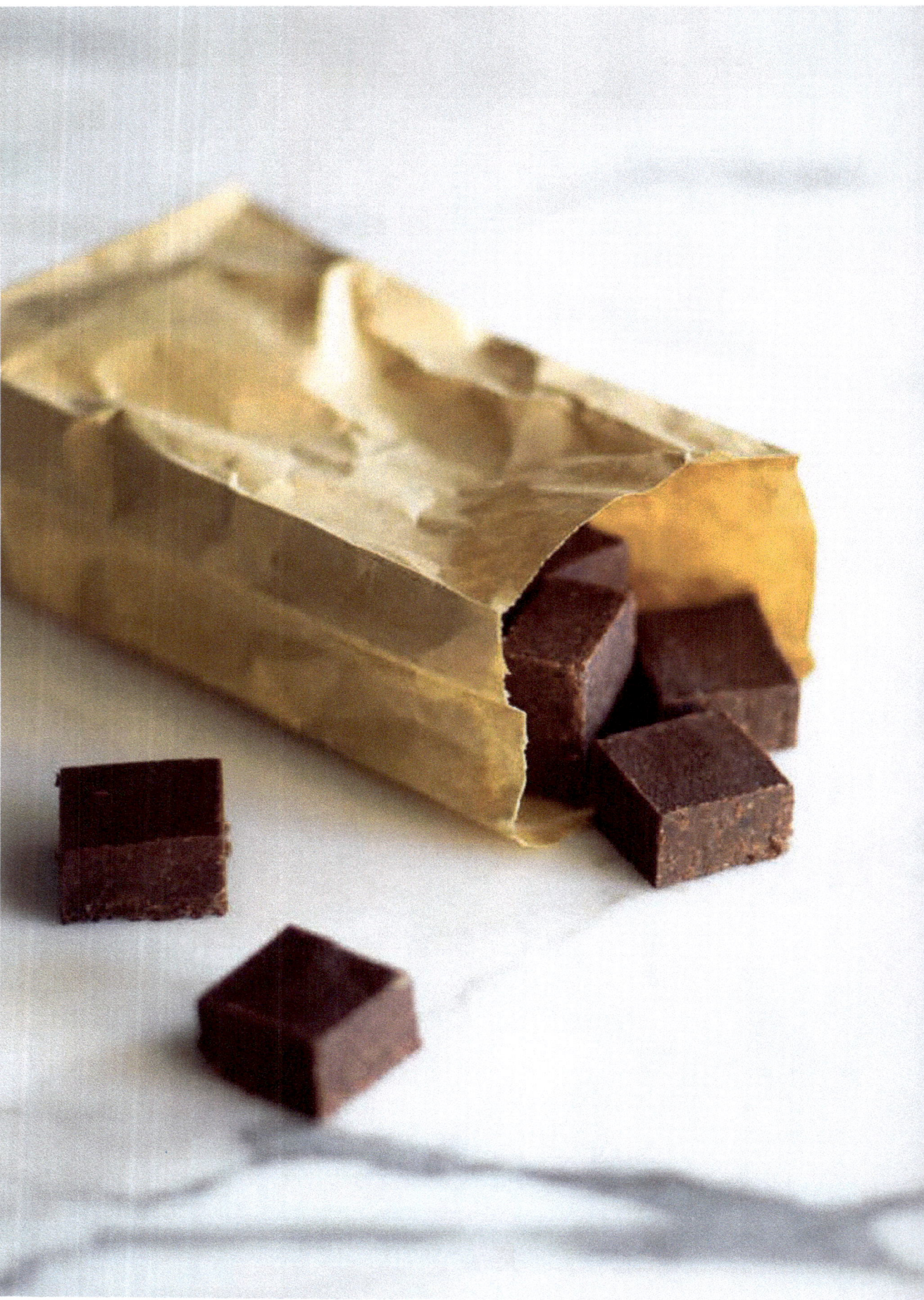

Hemp and Almond Ginger Lime Fudge

Hemp seeds are a complete protein, containing essential fats, vitamins and enzymes. They are a potent little superfood and can help with supporting optimal health, and when paired with the bright flavours of ginger and lime, they are a total winner.

Line a small ceramic baking dish with greaseproof paper. Place the almonds and hemp seeds in a food processor or Thermomix, and blitz in brief spurts so it forms a crumble texture, scraping down the sides in between (**TM** speed 5, 60 seconds). Set the crumble aside. In a double boiler, melt the cacao butter and coconut oil (**TM** 50 degrees, speed 2, 3 minutes), and then add in cacao powder, cacao nibs, maple syrup, vanilla paste, cayenne pepper, salt and essential oils and mix well (**TM** reverse speed 3, 45 seconds).

Press the fudge slice into your lined dish using a scrunched up piece of greaseproof paper initially, then with the back of a spoon to smooth out and refrigerate for one hour or until set.

Ingredients
1 cup (130g) almonds
1/3 cup (45g) hemp seeds
1/2 cup (60g) cacao butter
3 tbsp coconut oil
1/2 cup (50g) organic cacao powder
2 tbsp cacao nibs
3 tbsp (45g) maple syrup
1/4 tsp cayenne pepper
5 drops food-grade lime essential oil
5 drops food-grade ginger essential oil
1 tsp vanilla paste
Good pinch of pink salt

Damiana-infused Cacao Chocolates

This recipe is quite unique in that I feel it has a lot of alchemy in the mix. Damiana is a beautiful herb that has been used (historically) as an aphrodisiac and relaxant, and when combined with cinnamon, cacao and medicinal mushrooms – WOW! I feel that each time I make these that their energy deserves something special, so I brush gold dust into the chocolate moulds to really elevate them. You can buy damiana leaves dried from health food shops, and they also make a great tea.

Place a set of chocolate moulds on a baking tray. To make an infused butter, add the cacao butter and damiana to a small saucepan and put on low heat for 45 minutes to an hour, or in the **TM** on heat 50, speed 2. When your butter is ready, strain it through a fine sieve into a separate jug.

Using a glass bowl or a Thermomix, add the strained cacao butter and all other ingredients and mix thoroughly to create a smooth chocolate batter (**TM** speed 3, 2 minutes).

Pour into moulds, refrigerate for one hour or until set. Devour, savouring the flavour and effects.

NOTE I use a medicinal mushroom blend of chaga, reishi, cordyceps, lion's mane, shiitake, mitake, and poria. Medicinal mushroom blends are available at health food shops.

1 cup (120g) cacao butter
1/3 cup dried damiana leaves
1 cup (100g) organic cacao powder
1/3 cup (60g) coconut oil
4 tbsp (60g) maple syrup
2 tsp medicinal mushroom powder
1 tsp maca powder
1/2 tsp spirulina powder
2 drops food-grade copaiba essential oil
3 drops food-grade cinnamon essential oil
Pinch of pink salt

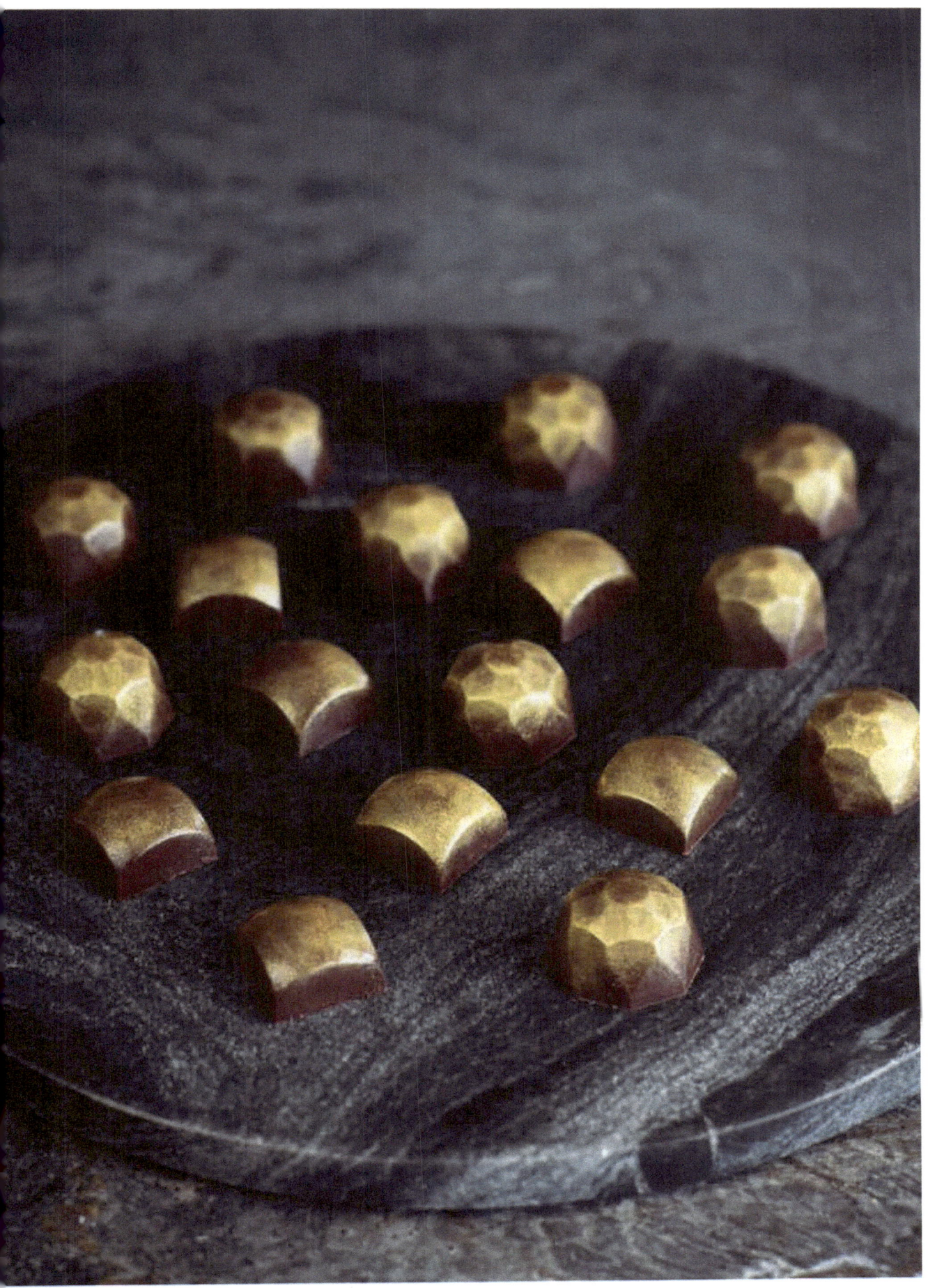

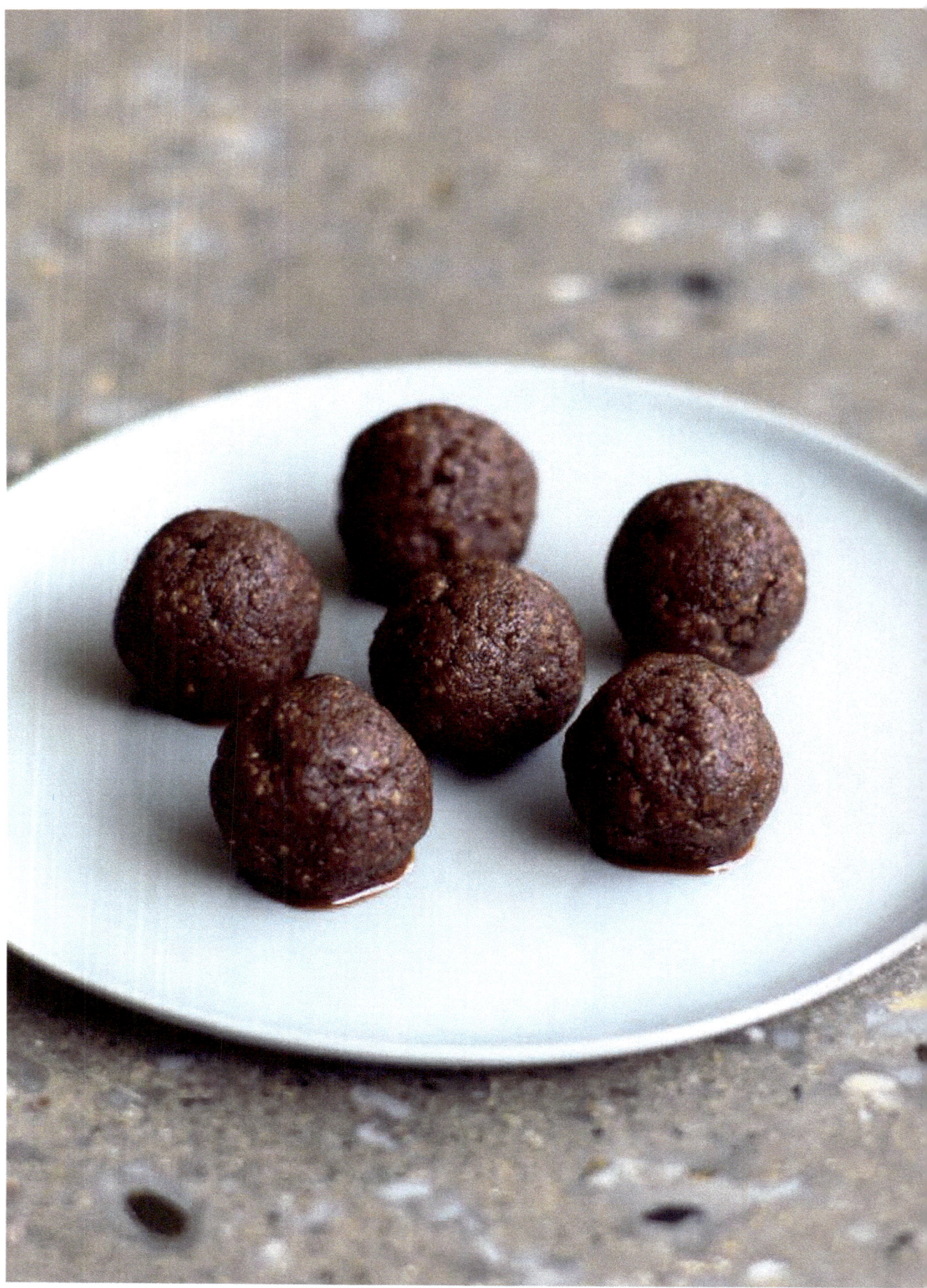

Fer-RAW-Ro Cacao Bliss Balls

The flavour of toasted hazelnuts is so delicious and this simple bliss ball recipe has many nourishing foods that keep you satisfied for hours and hours.

Line a tray or plate with greaseproof paper. In a large frypan over medium heat, add the hazelnut meal and stir continuously until fragrant and becoming golden in colour. Pour the meal into your food processor, or Thermomix. Add the remaining ingredients and blend (**TM** speed 7) until well combined and resembling a fine sticky crumble. Use your hands to press and shape the mixture into balls. Place on tray and set in the refrigerator for one hour or until set.

- 2 cups (260g) hazelnut meal
- 12 Medjool dates, pitted
- 2 tbsp maple syrup
- 1 tbsp hemp seeds
- 3 tbsp organic cacao powder
- 1 tsp coconut butter, melted
- 1 tsp maca powder
- 5 drops food-grade lemon essential oil

Spiced Cashew Chia Fudge

I love to include cinnamon in my treats – aside from its lovely warming nature, it can help to support healthy blood sugar levels. Cassia has a similar flavour profile to cinnamon.

Line a baking tray with greaseproof paper. In a double boiler over low heat, melt the cacao butter and coconut oil, stir to combine (**TM** heat 50, speed 2, 5 minutes). Add all other ingredients and mix well (**TM** reverse speed 2, don't chop, you want the whole cashew effect when slicing and serving). Spread out onto tray, press down evenly, then sprinkle turmeric coconut on top and refrigerate for approximately one hour, or until set. Cut into squares and serve.

- 1 cup (120g) cacao butter
- ¼ cup (45g) coconut oil
- ½ cup (50g) organic cacao powder
- ¼ cup (70g) maple syrup
- 2 tbsp hemp seeds
- Pinch of pink salt
- ¼ cup (40g) chia seeds
- 1 cup (130g) cashews
- 1 tsp lucuma powder
- 2 drops food-grade cinnamon essential oil
- 1 drop food-grade cassia essential oil
- ½ cup shredded coconut, coloured with ½ tsp of turmeric

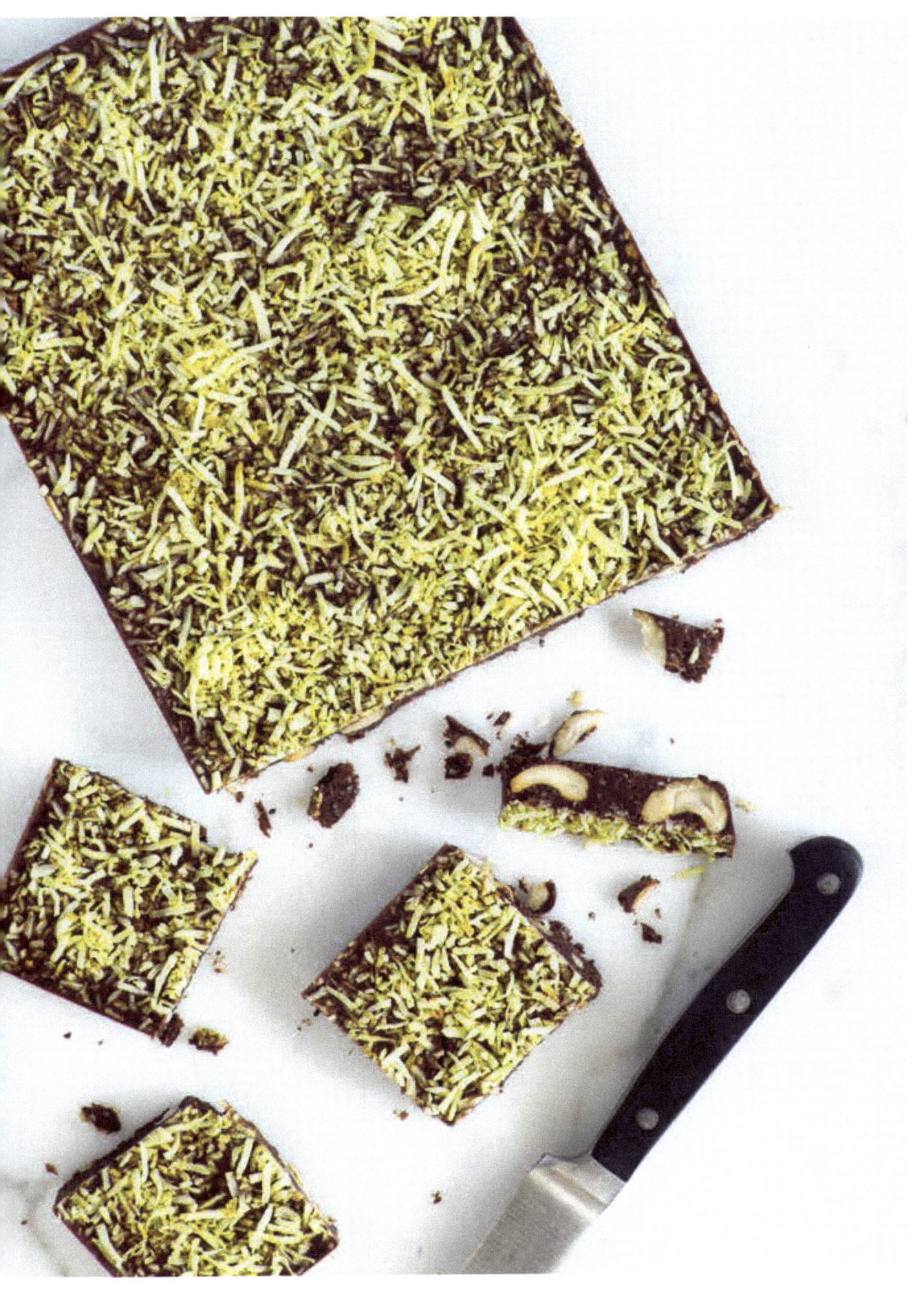

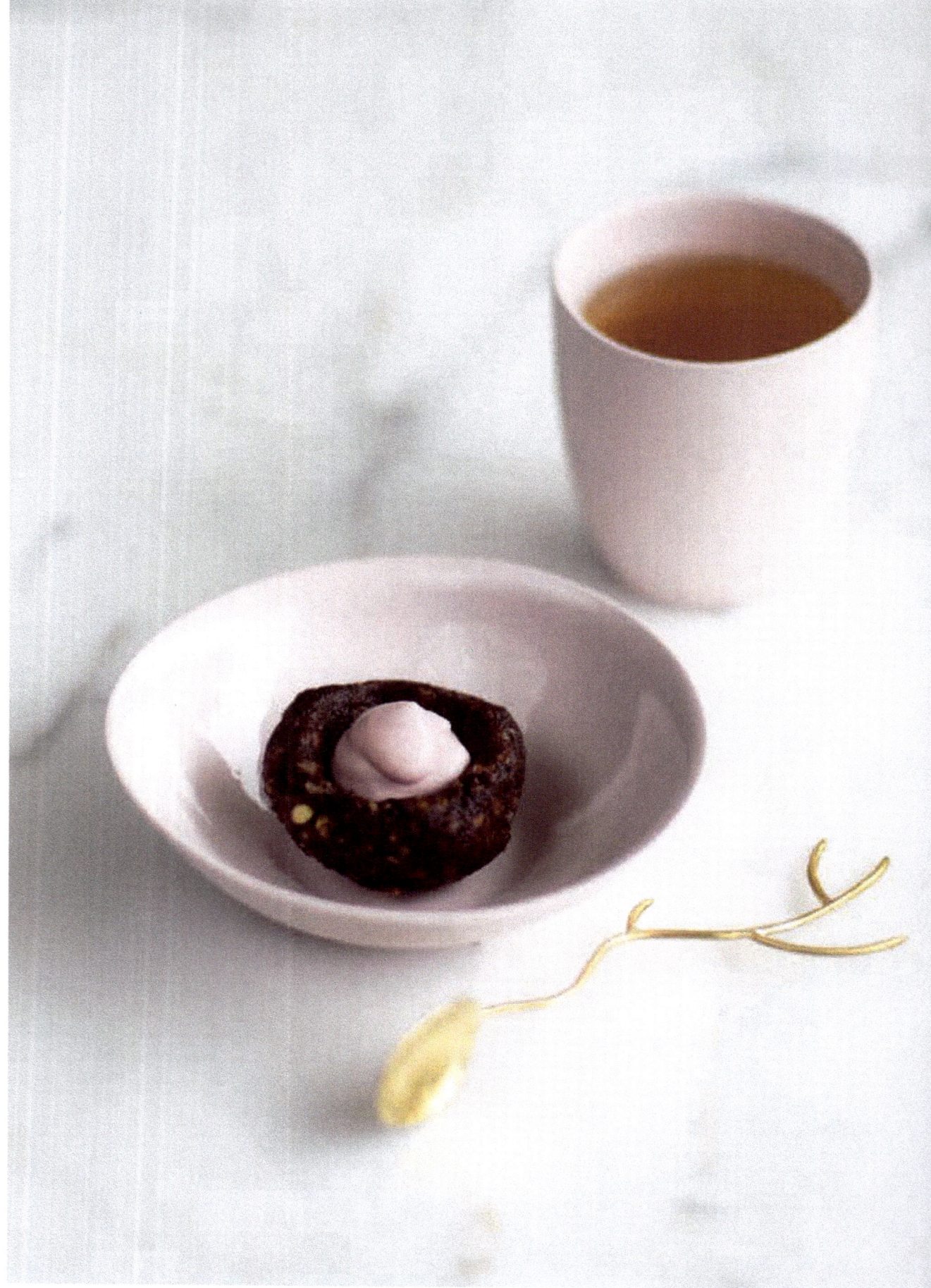

Nuts and Seeds Chunky Pods with Coconut Cream

These might seem a little more fiddly than some of the other recipes, but I promise you they are a delightful-looking dessert and truly worth it.

To make the pod base: Place all base ingredients in a food processor or Thermomix. Roughly blend everything together until it resembles a crumble mixture (**TM** speed 6, 2 minutes). Roll into small balls, then, like you are making a pinch pot, use your thumb and fingers to make a small well in each ball. Refrigerate while making the coconut cream.

To make the whipped coconut cream, scoop out the top level of thickened coconut cream from the tin into a glass bowl. Add beetroot powder, coconut paste and orange oil, then whip with hand mixer for a few minutes. When it starts to thicken, add maple syrup and salt and whip for a short blast to mix in. Refrigerate for 20 minutes, then add a dollop to your pods. Return the pods to the fridge to set for 45 minutes to an hour.

NOTES The pod mixture will stick to your hands a little, so after making a few pods give them a wash to make them easier to handle.

BASE

2 cups (260g) assorted nuts and seeds (eg. sesame, sunflower, almonds, walnuts, hemp, pecan, poppy)

10 Medjool dates, pitted

2 tbsp maple syrup

3 tbsp coconut oil

3 tbsp activated buckinis

1/3 cup (35g) organic cacao powder

1 tsp medicinal mushroom powder (I like the SuperFeast brand)

1 tsp cinnamon powder

3 drops food-grade cardamom essential oil

Pinch of pink salt

COCONUT WHIPPED CREAM

400ml tin coconut cream (refrigerated for 2 hours)

1/3 tsp beetroot or blueberry powder (this is just for colour)

1 tbsp maple syrup

1 tsp vanilla paste

2 tbsp coconut paste

5 drops food-grade wild orange essential oil

Small pinch of pink salt, to thicken

Peppermint Hemp Balls

Peppermint essential oil is the perfect mid-afternoon pick me up when you are starting to feel a little tired, and when bound with all the goodness of nuts and seeds, it becomes a powerful way to get through the day.

Roughly chop the coating ingredients, then place in a bowl.

Line a tray with greaseproof paper. Place all ingredients in a food processor or Thermomix, blend well (**TM** speed 6, 60 seconds). If the mix seems dry, add a little coconut water. Roll into small balls and coat in the crumble mix, place on a tray then refrigerate for one hour or until set.

Any leftover crumb is a delicious boost for a smoothie!

1 cup (130g) activated almonds
1 cup (130g) activated walnuts
12 Medjool dates, pitted
1/3 cup (35g) goji berries
2 tbsp LSA (linseed, sunflower, almond)
2 tbsp chia seeds
2 tbsp coconut oil, melted
1 tbsp honey
3 tsp organic cacao powder
1 tsp blueberry powder
1/2 tsp cinnamon
1/4 cup (20g) hemp seeds
coconut water, if needed
4 drops food-grade peppermint essential oil

COATING

3 tbsp chia seeds
3 tbsp shredded coconut
3 tbsp almonds, chopped
3 tbsp goji berries, chopped
1 tsp maca powder
1 tbsp cacao nibs

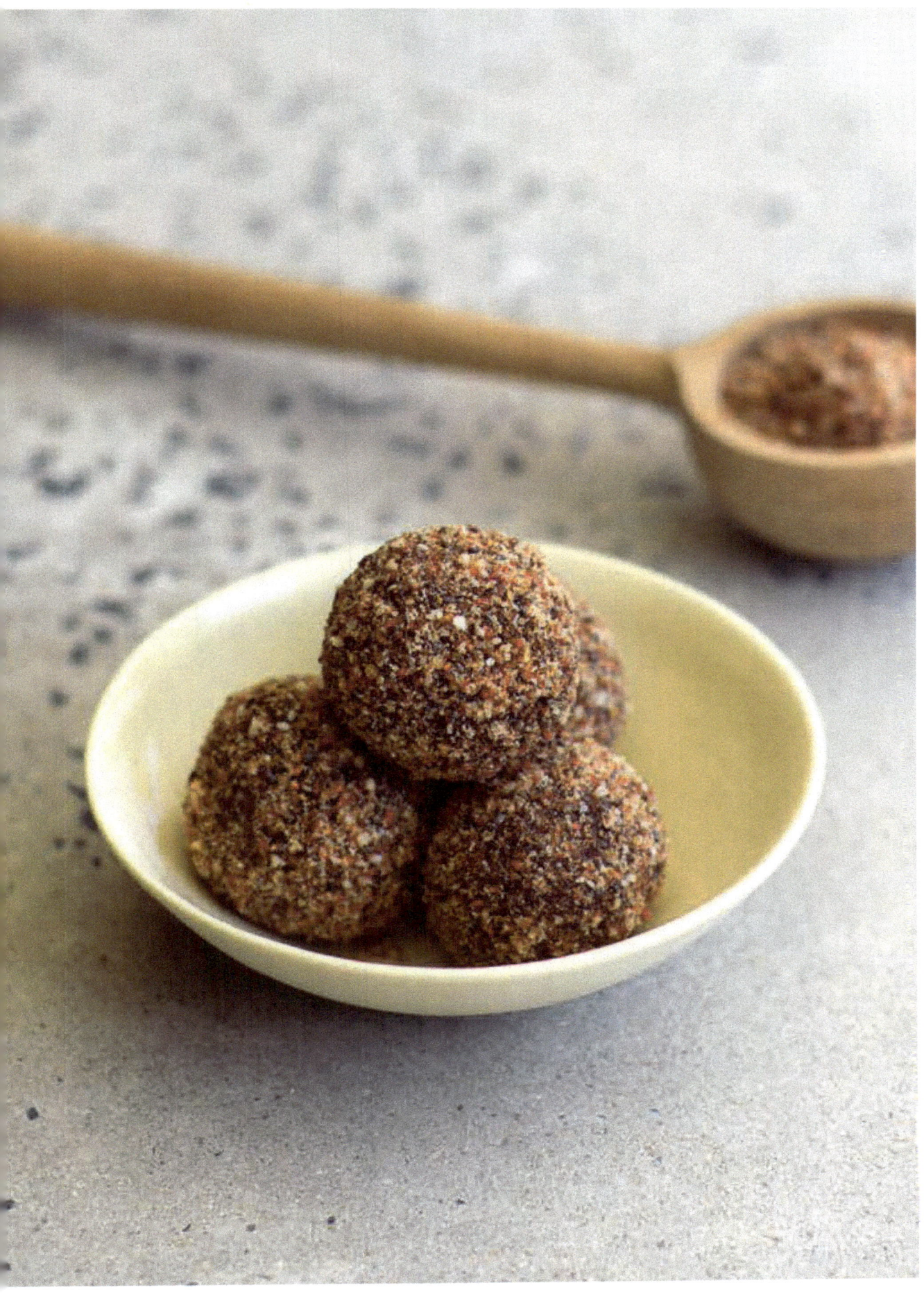

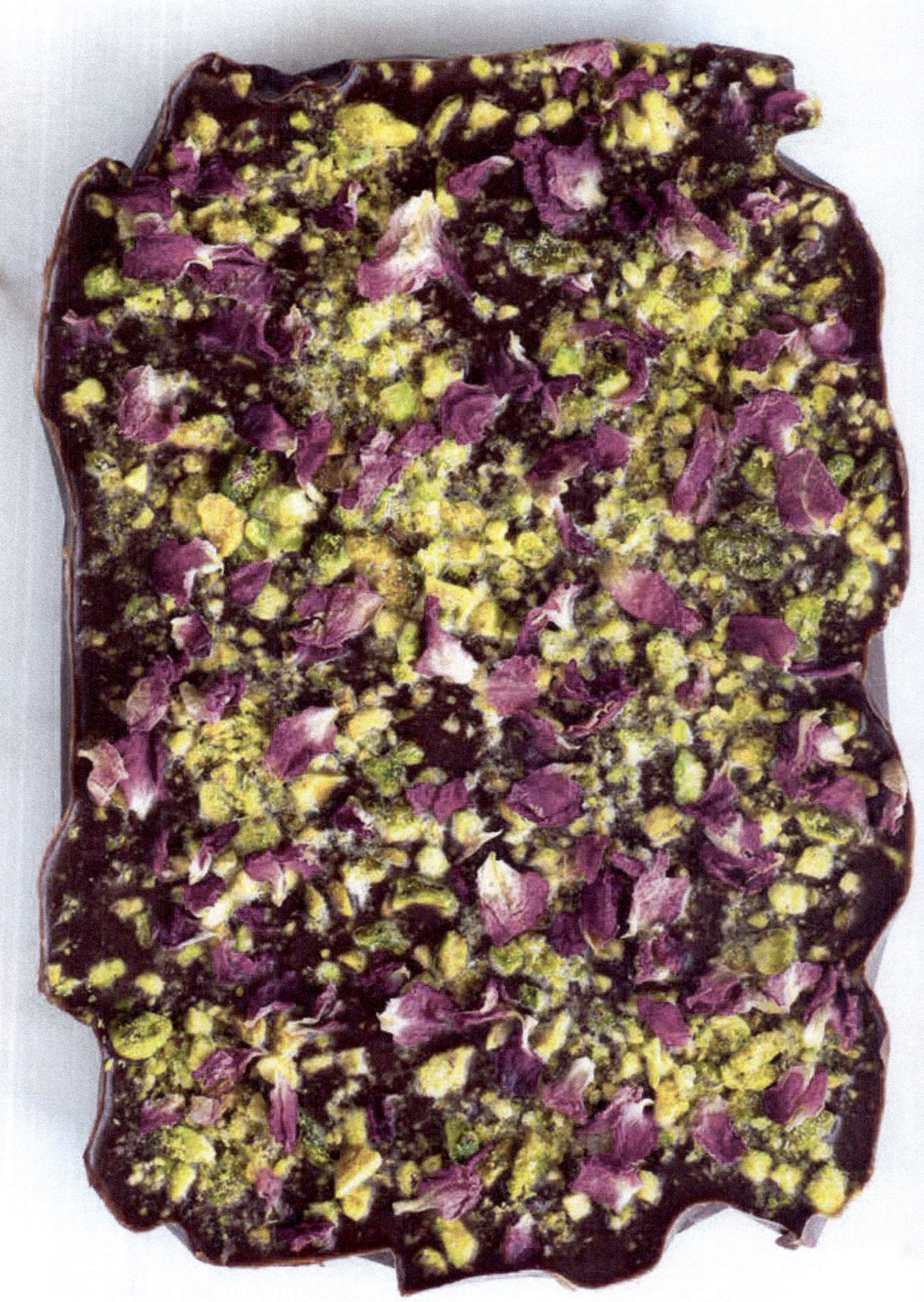

Raw Turkish Delight

This take on Turkish Delight has all the delightful fragrant notes you know and love from the original – rose, cinnamon and pistachio – plus some extra goodness thrown in.

Line a tray with greaseproof paper. In a medium size double boiler over low heat, melt the coconut oil (**TM** heat 50, speed 1, 60 seconds). If you aren't using a Thermomix, roughly chop the pistachios, coconut and dried fruit together. Add all remaining ingredients (except extra pistachios and rose petals) to your saucepan or Thermomix, and mix together (**TM** slightly chop, speed 4 for 20 seconds).

Pour evenly onto tray, smooth out and garnish with chopped pistachios and rose petals. Refrigerate for one hour or until set.

Ingredients
¾ cup (135g) coconut oil
¼ cup (15g) shredded coconut
½ cup (65g) pistachios, plus extra for topping
¼ cup cranberries and goji berries (60g total)
2 tbsp crystallized ginger, chopped
½ cup (50g) organic cacao powder
¼ cup (70g) maple syrup
½ tsp ground cinnamon
1 tsp vanilla paste
1 drop food-grade rose essential oil
5 drops food-grade wild orange essential oil
Pinch of pink salt
Edible rose petals

Honey and Bee Pollen Lemon Chocolates

I am bee mad, so when I found some really cute moulds of bees and hives on eBay, I knew I had to create a healthy chocolate showcasing the benefits of pollen and raw honey. To make them extra adorable, I used gold dust to highlight their little bodies. (#savethebees)

Set a silicone chocolate mould on a baking tray. In a double boiler over low heat, melt the cacao butter and coconut oil together (**TM** heat 50, 5 minutes, speed 2). Then add all other ingredients in and mix well until all is blended smoothly. Spoon into moulds and refrigerate until set, approximately one hour. They should pop out easily once set.

1 cup (120g) cacao butter
¾ cup (75g) organic cacao powder
2 tbsp coconut oil
2 tbsp raw honey
2 tsp bee pollen
Pinch of salt
5 drops food-grade lemon essential oil

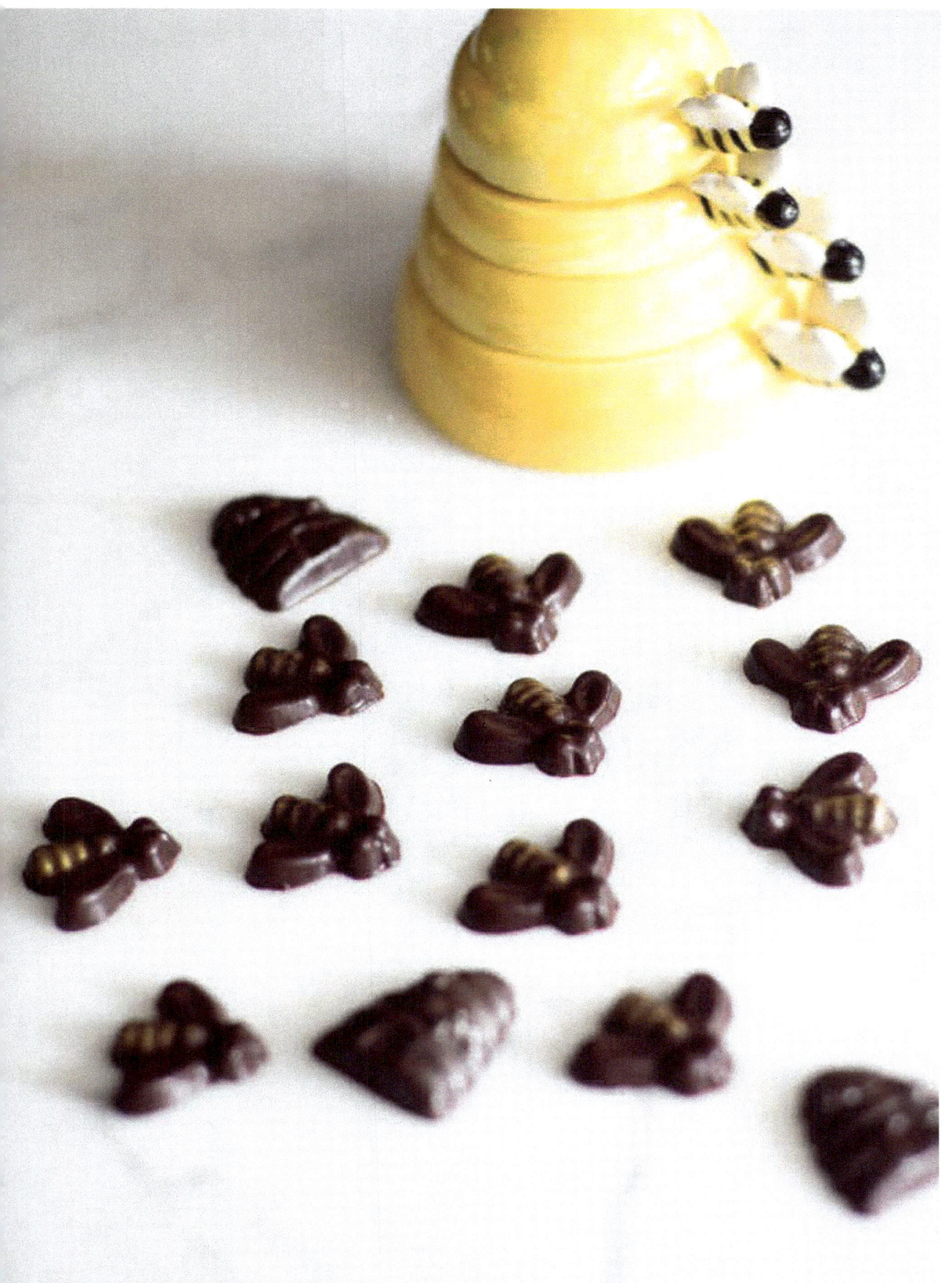

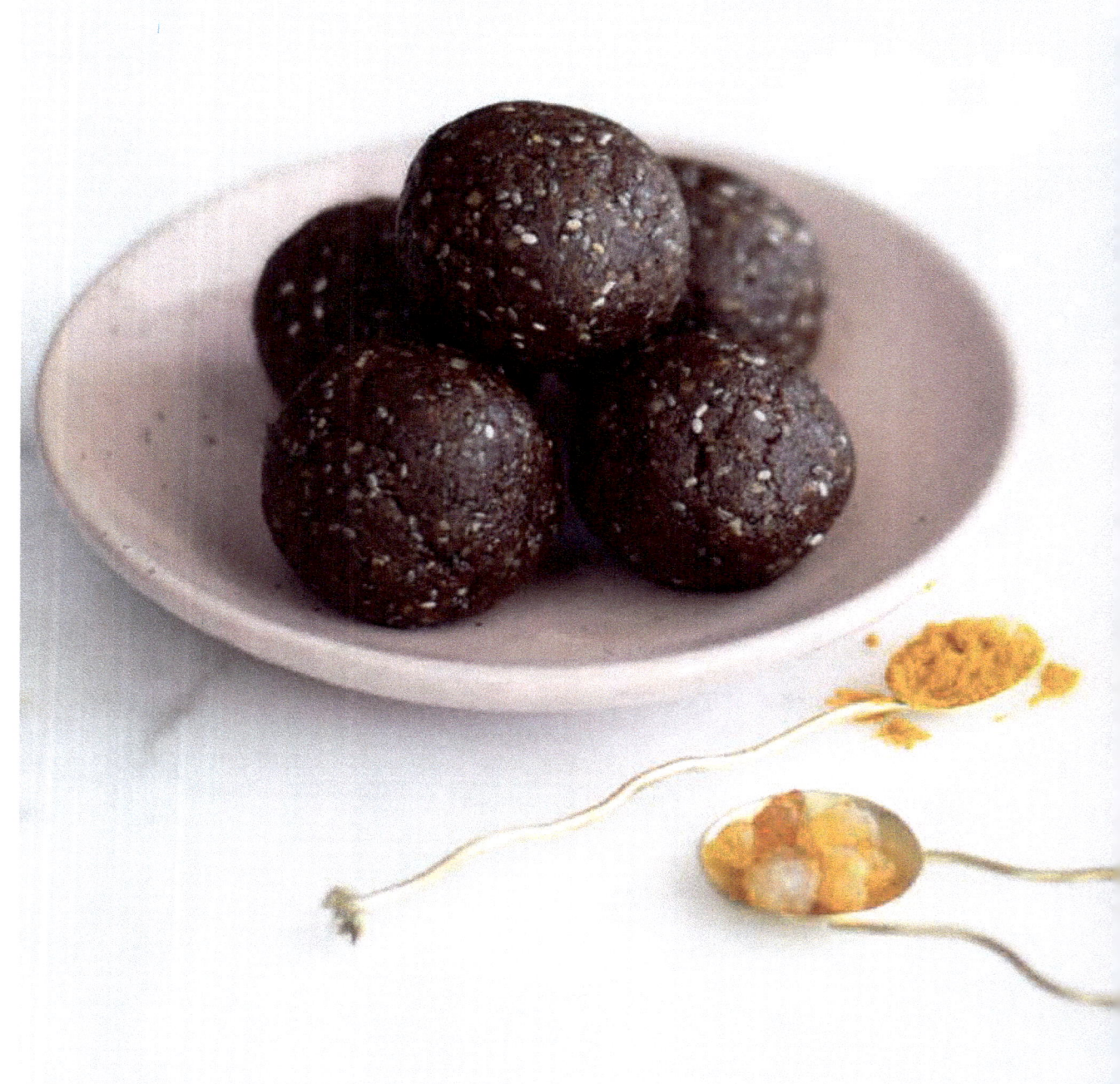

Three Wise Men Bliss Balls

I fell in love with the idea of creating a snack that embodied gold, frankincense and myrrh – surely something so potent could only be amazing. With the incredible health benefits of turmeric combined with a collection of superfood powders, cacao, seeds, and myrrh and frankincense essential oils, they really are a gift!

Line a baking tray with greaseproof paper. Blitz everything well in a food processor or Thermomix (**TM** speed 7) and roll into even sized balls. Place balls on tray and refrigerate for 45 minutes to one hour or until set.

TIP Roll balls in large circles to make even circular shapes. Wipe excess walnut oil off in between rolling a few.

- 2 cups (260g) walnuts
- 1 cup (130g) almonds
- ½ cup (30g) shredded coconut
- 10 Medjool dates, pitted
- 4 tbsp coconut oil
- 4 tbsp sunflower seeds
- 2 tbsp chia seeds
- 2-3 tbsp maple syrup
- 4 tbsp (30g) organic cacao powder
- 1 tbsp maca powder
- 1 tsp organic turmeric powder
- 1 tsp medicinal mushrooms powder
- 4 drops food-grade myrrh essential oil
- 8 drops food-grade frankincense essential oil
- Pinch of pink salt

Fruit Nut Seed Clusters

This is a healthy variation to the chocolate crackle, without the sugar overload and comedown, combining nuts, seeds and some special Inca berries for a really lush textural combination.

Set roughly 20 paper patty pans on a baking tray. To make the nut and seed mix: Roughly chop dried fruit, nuts and pepitas, or if using a Thermomix, chop on speed 5 for 10 seconds.

Add remaining ingredients and mix through well (**TM** reverse speed 3), then place a heaped teaspoon-sized amount into patty tins, lightly pressing them together to hold shape. Refrigerate for 15 minutes.

To make the raw chocolate: In a small double boiler over low heat, or in a Thermomix, melt cacao butter and coconut oil together (**TM** heat 50, speed 2, 5 minutes) and then mix in all other ingredients well. Spoon the chocolate mixture into each patty tin covering well and refrigerate for 30 minutes or until set.

NUT AND SEED MIX

1½ cups (195g) almonds
1 cup (130g) pecans
⅓ cup (40g) pepitas
½ cup (80g) sun muscats
½ cup (65g) dried apricots
¼ cup (35g) Inca berries
⅓ cup (20g) shredded coconut
¼ cup (25g) hemp seeds
3 tbsp of cacao nibs
3 tbsp maple syrup
2 tbsp coconut oil
2 tbsp black sesame seeds
1 tsp acai powder

RAW CHOCOLATE

½ cup (60g) cacao butter
⅓ cup (60g) coconut oil
½ cup (50g) organic cacao powder
¼ cup (70g) maple syrup
pinch of pink salt
8 drops food-grade wild orange essential oil
4 drops food-grade cinnamon essential oil

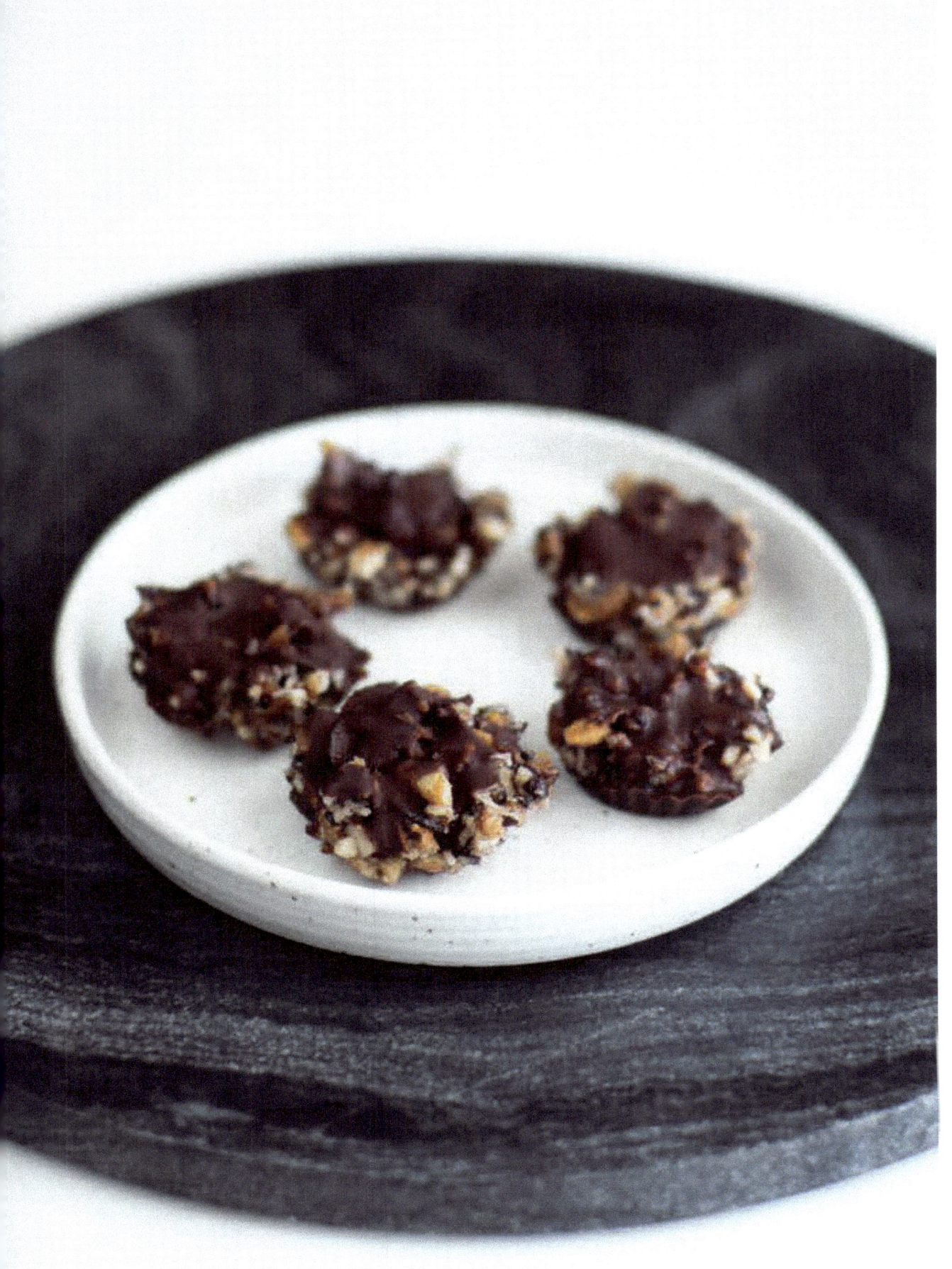

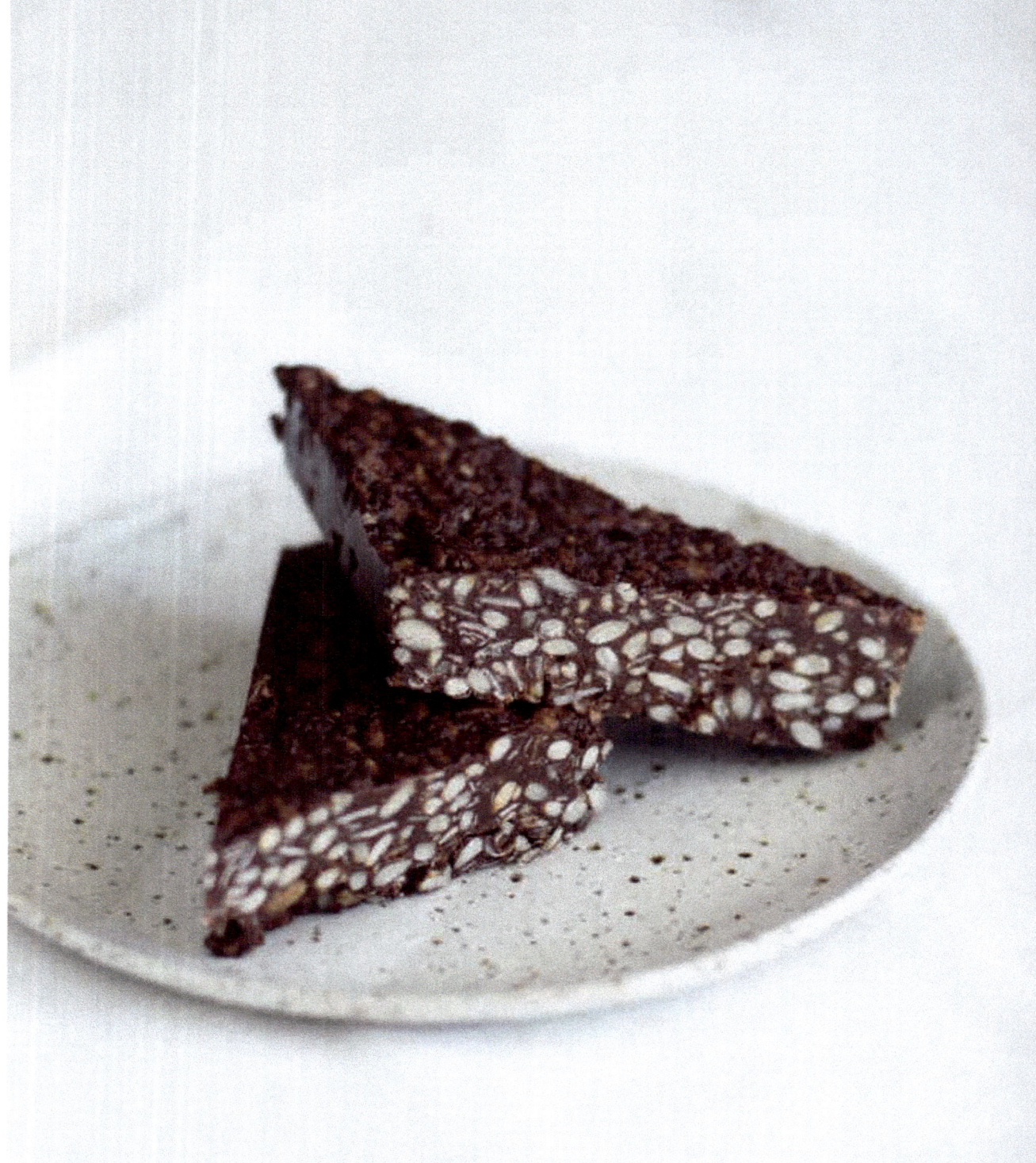

Lemon Coconut Rough

A lemon coconut rough is the stuff of nostalgia, but here I have swapped all the usual suspects of sugar, flour and egg for densely nutritious and delicious ingredients.

Line a baking tray with greaseproof paper. In a frypan over medium heat, slowly dry toast the sunflower seeds. Remove from pan and set aside. Add in shredded coconut to the same pan and toast lightly. Set aside in a bowl to cool.

In a small double boiler over low heat or in a Thermomix, melt cacao butter and coconut oil together (**TM** heat 50, speed 2, 5 minutes). Add all other ingredients including the toasted seeds and coconut, ,and mix well (**TM** reverse speed 3, don't chop).

Spread mix onto tray evenly, pressing down, and top with coconut flakes, then refrigerate for one hour or until set. Crack into chunks and serve.

- 2 cups (300g) sunflower seeds
- 2 cups (130g) shredded coconut
- 1 cup (120g) cacao butter
- 1/3 cup (60g) coconut oil
- 3/4 cup (75g) organic cacao powder
- 1 cup (130g) walnuts (chopped finely)
- 1/4 cup (70g) maple syrup
- 1 heaped tbsp finely grated lemon rind
- 1 tsp vanilla paste
- 3 drops food-grade cinnamon essential oil
- Pinch of pink salt

Macadamia Fudge with Limoncello Ganache

For a decadent fudge treat, this macadamia slab is so delicious and is topped off with the addition of a limoncello ganache, representing my love for the Italian lifestyle and culture.

Line a baking tray with greaseproof paper. In a food processor or Thermomix, blend together the dates, coconut and macadamias to form a crumble, then and add all other ingredients in and mix well. It will require a few times of scraping and mixing, as the consistency is quite fudge like (**TM** speed 7, 2 minutes). Scrape mixture onto lined tray, pressing down evenly and firmly. Set aside.

For the ganache, in a small double boiler over low heat, melt the coconut oil (**TM** heat 37, speed 1, 2 minutes). Add all other ingredients except the limoncello and mix. Add limoncello in slowly, mixing as you go. Spread ganache over the slice. Sprinkle the cacao nibs over the top and refrigerate for one hour or until set.

FUDGE BASE

2 cups (260g) macadamia nuts

2 cups (130g) shredded coconut

10 Medjool dates, pitted

¾ cup (75g) organic cacao powder

¼ cup (70g) organic maple syrup

1 tsp acai powder

3 drops food-grade cardamom essential oil

Pinch of pink salt

GANACHE

¼ cup (50g) coconut oil

⅓ cup (90g) maple syrup

½ cup (50g) organic cacao powder

8 drops food-grade lemon essential oil

5 tbsp limoncello… from Bellagio, Italy of course!

Pinch of pink salt

¼ cup (30g) raw cacao nibs, for topping

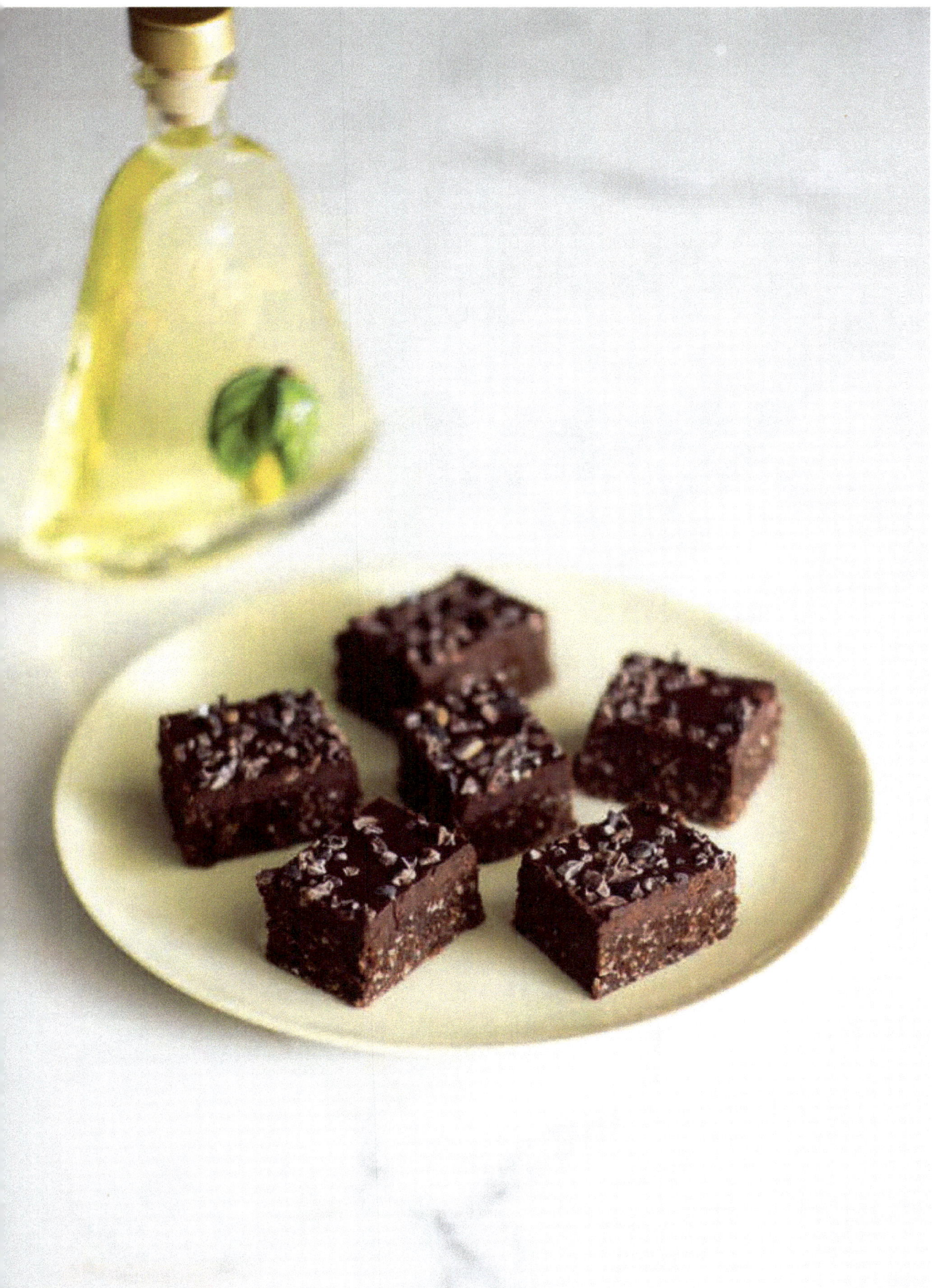

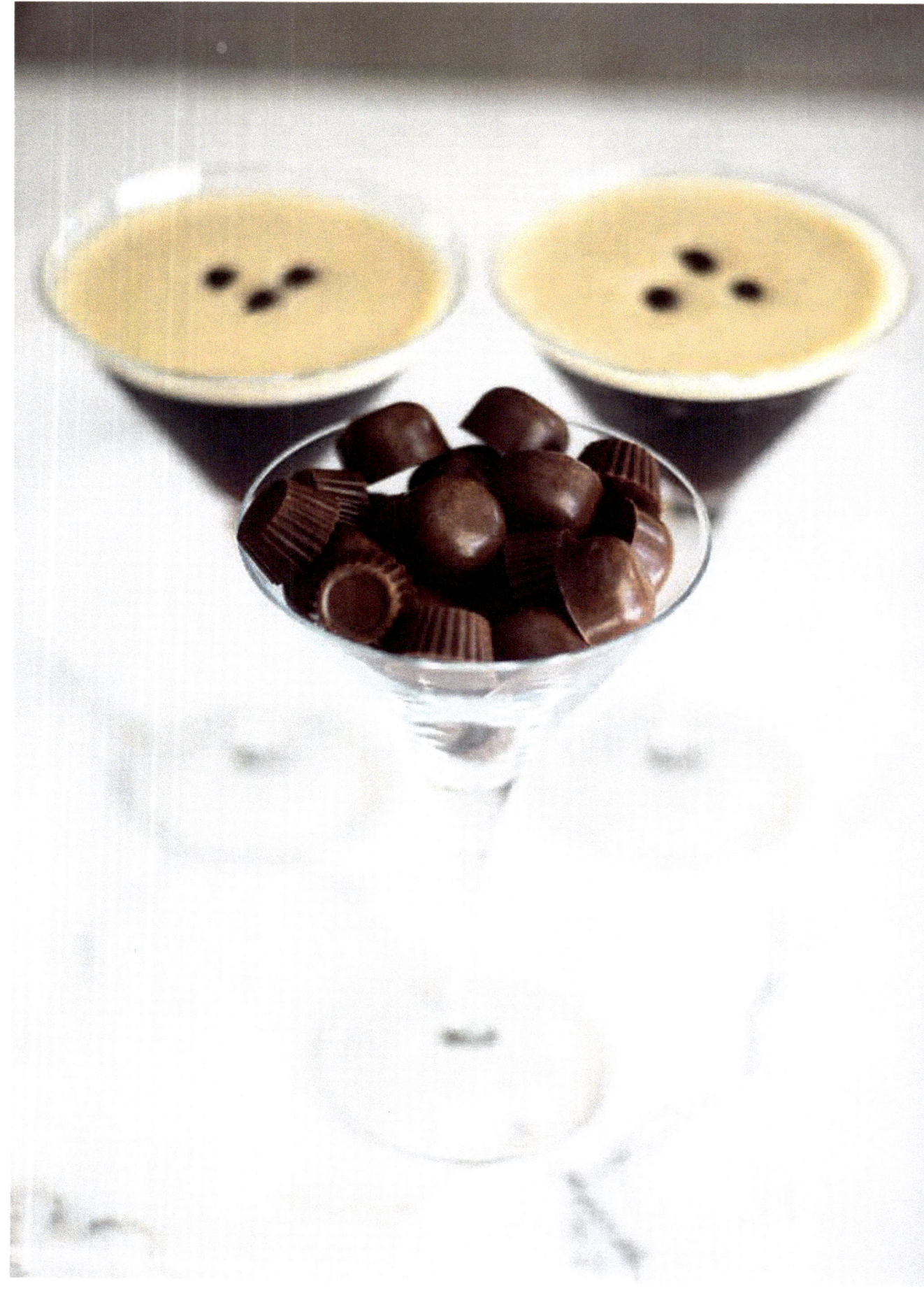

Espresso martini chocolates

Our signature Friday night cocktail bit of fun, adapted into a chocolate treat.

Melt cacao butter and coconut oil first on low heat (**TM** heat 50, speed 2, 5 minutes) or using the double boiler method. Then add in cacao powder, maple syrup and salt, mixing well to form a smooth glossy batter.

Once the basic chocolate mix is ready, slowly mix in a 15ml shot each of three different alcohols and of espresso coffee. Mix well.

Spoon or pour into chocolate moulds and refrigerate until set, approximately one hour.

TIP Have all the measures of alcohol and coffee prepared together in a jug, to make it easy to add slowly while mixing the chocolate.

HEADING

1 cup (120g) cacao butter
¼ cup (45g) coconut oil
1 cup (100g) organic cacao powder
¼ cup (70g) maple syrup
Pinch of pink salt
15ml Kahlua
15ml vanilla vodka
15ml Creme de Cacao
15ml espresso coffee

Turkish Delight Minis

This is a completely charming sweet to wow your guests at your next dinner party. These mini Turkish Delights look so appealing as a bite-sized morsel with a tuft of Persian fairy floss on top.

Set roughly 20 paper patty pans on a baking tray. In a bowl, mix together all the ingredients (except for the toppings) until smooth and glossy. Spoon a small amount into each patty tin.

While chocolate is still liquid, garnish each with pistachios and rose petals. Refrigerate for 45 minutes to one hour, or until set, then place some Persian fairy floss on each and serve.

TIP You can buy edible rose petals and Persian fairy floss from food stores and quality supermarkets.

BASE

1 cup (180g) coconut oil, melted

¾ cup (75g) organic cacao powder

¼ cup (70g) maple syrup

Pinch of pink salt

½ tsp ground cinnamon

1 tsp vanilla paste

¾ cup (95g) pistachios, chopped

½ cup (65g) hazelnuts, chopped

¼ cup (15g) shredded coconut

¾ cup (100g total) cranberries and goji berries, chopped

3 tbsp crystallized ginger, chopped

1 tsp maca powder

1 drop food-grade rose essential oil

3 drops food-grade cardamom essential oil

3 drops food-grade cinnamon essential oil

8 drops Food-grade wild orange essential oil

TOPPING

Crushed edible rose petals

Persian fairy floss

Pistachios, chopped

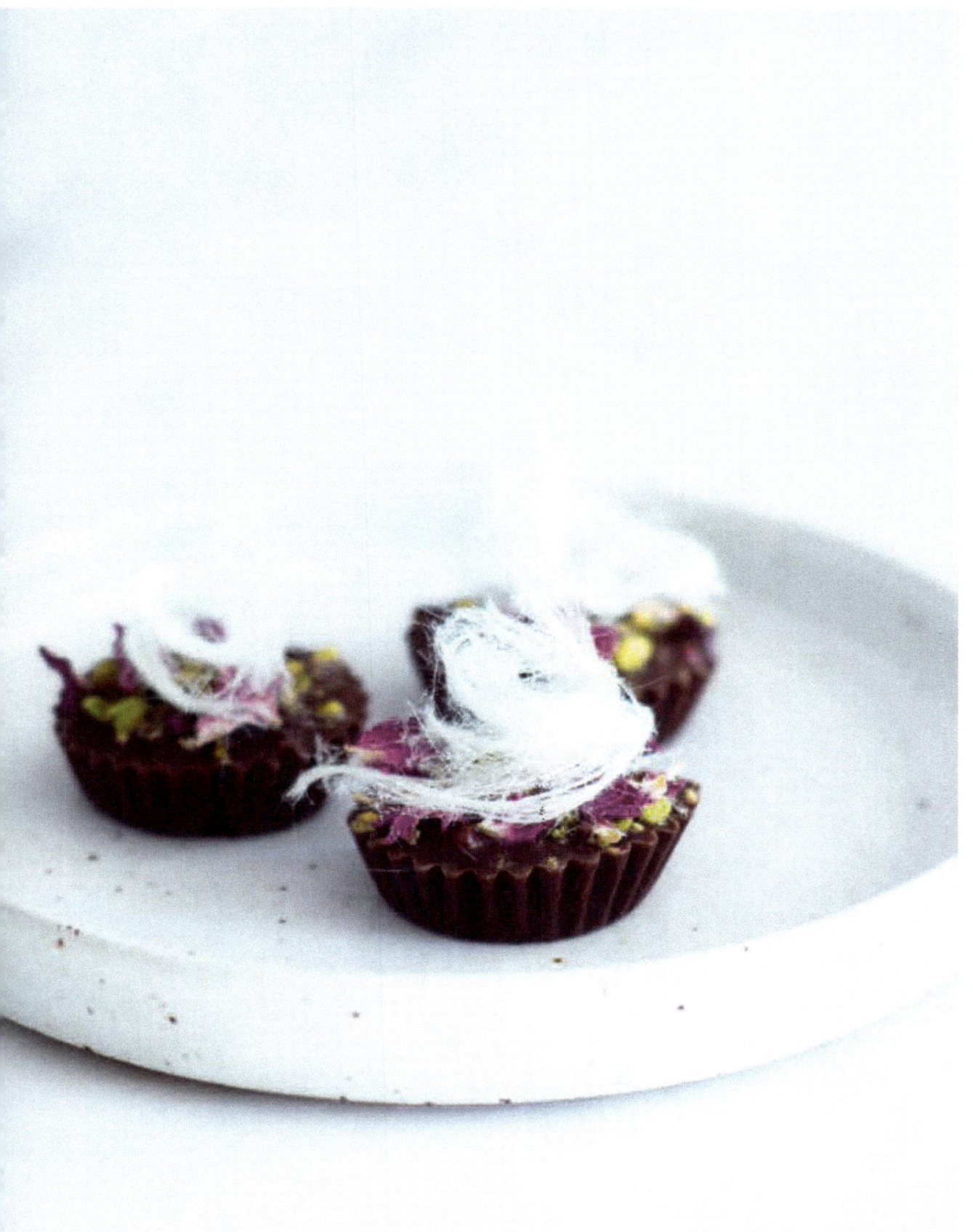

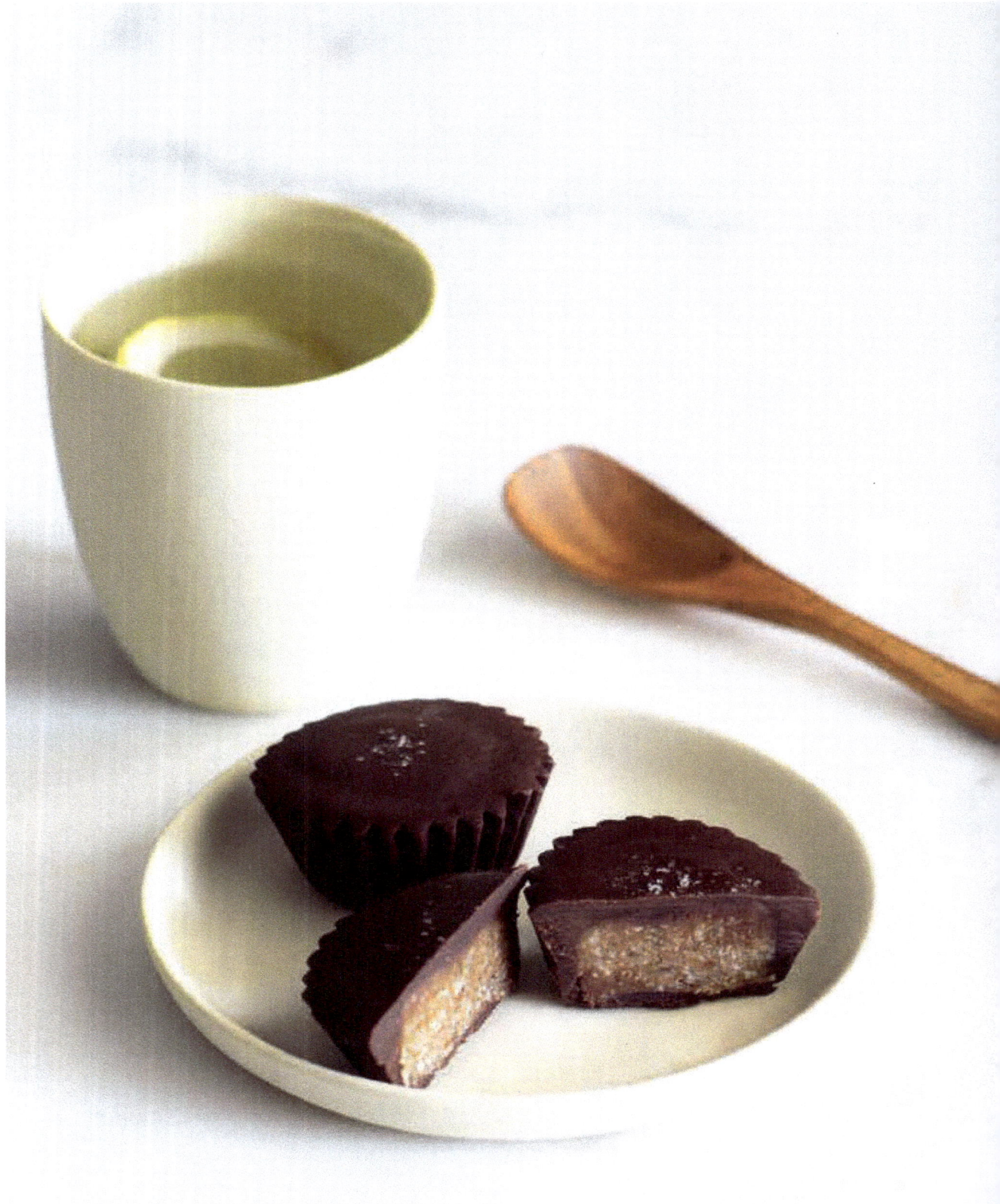

Salted Caramel Soft Centre Chocolates

Creating an easy and healthy soft caramel, with dates and coconut, as opposed to the truckload of sugar and additives!

Set around 20-30 small paper patty pans on a baking tray. In a food processor or Thermomix, blitz all the ingredients for the caramel filling very well until it forms a caramel consistency (**TM** speed 7, 60 seconds).

In a small saucepan over low heat or in a Thermomix, melt the cacao butter and coconut oil together (**TM** heat 50, speed 2, 5 minutes), then add in other ingredients, mixing until smooth. Add a small amount to the patty pans to form a base, spreading up the sides of the pans. While chocolate is still liquified, add a small coin-sized disc of caramel mixture to each. Lastly add more chocolate to seal the mixture, and refrigerate for one hour or until set.

TIP With the sea salt garnish, allow the chocolates to start to set and place a flake or two on each top, so they don't sink into the chocolate.

RAW CARAMEL FILLING

12 Medjool dates, pitted

2 cups (130g) shredded coconut

2 tsp chia seeds

1 tsp vanilla paste

½ tsp pink salt

RAW CHOCOLATE MIX

1 cup of cacao butter (120g)

¼ cup of coconut oil (45g)

1 cup of organic cacao powder (100g)

¼ cup of maple syrup (70g)

1 tsp maca powder

12 drops food-grade wild orange essential oil

Pinch of pink salt

Sea salt flakes, to garnish

Cacao Elixir

When I have a mindfulness or meditation group to facilitate, I find this tonic really assists in opening the heart and stilling the mind. Cacao has been used in ceremonies for centuries as a tonic to bring the mind, body and spirit back into balance. With the addition of the other ingredients it is such a healing elixir.

Place all ingredient in a medium saucepan over medium heat, or into your Thermomix bowl. Heat to a slow simmer for 10 minutes, whisking all the time (**TM** heat 50, speed 4, 8-10 minutes). Pour into small glasses to serve.

400ml tin coconut milk
½ cup (50g) organic cacao powder
¼ cup (70g) maple syrup
3 tbsp cacao butter
1 tbsp coconut butter
1 tsp turmeric
1 tsp maca powder
¼ tsp cayenne pepper
1 drop food-grade cinnamon essential oil
1 drop food-grade cardamom essential oil
2 drops food-grade wild orange essential oil
1 drop food-grade rose essential oil
Pinch of pink salt
1 cup of water

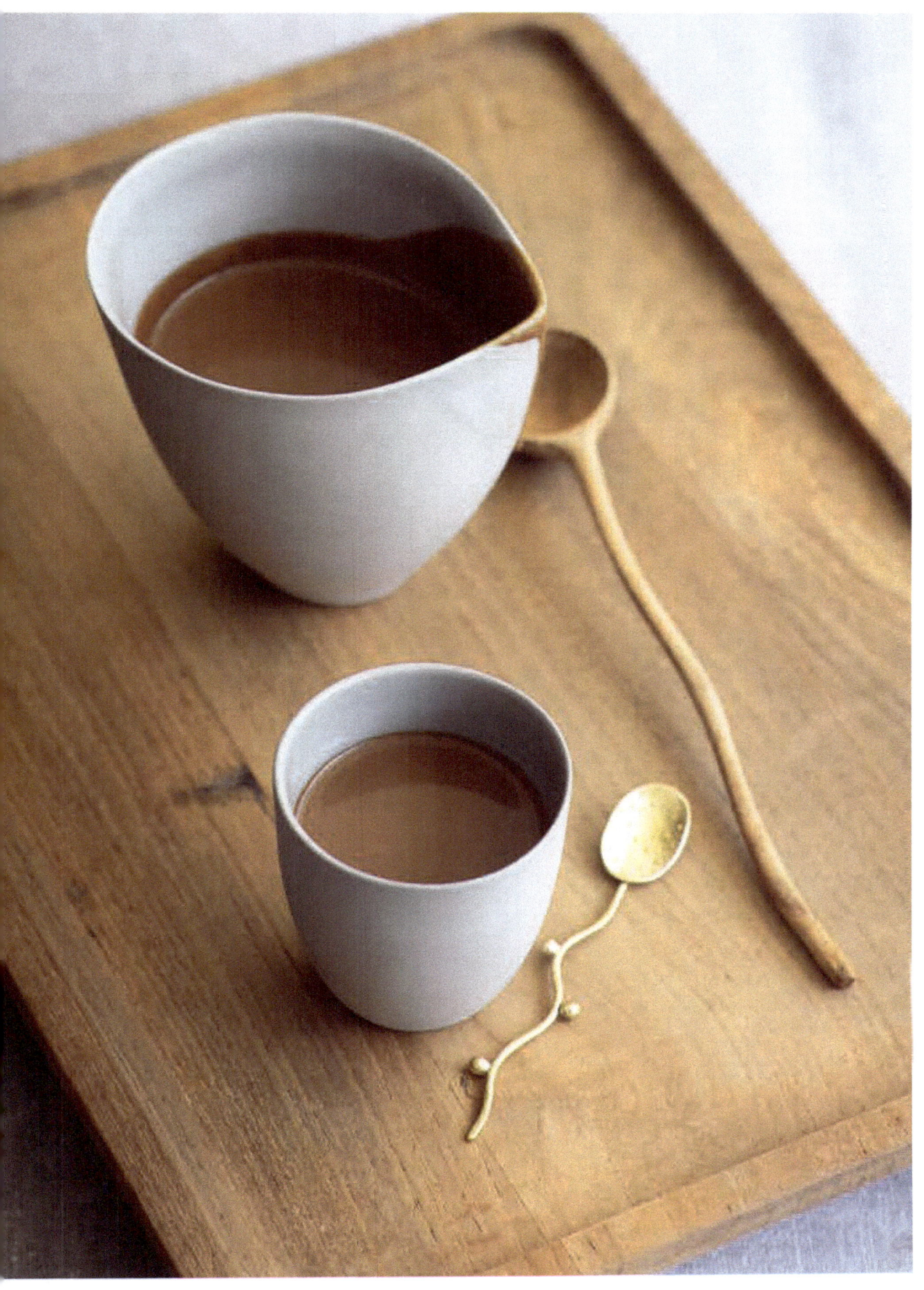

Drinks

One or two ice blocks can be added to any of these juices and smoothies. Blitz on high in your food processor Thermomix for at least one minute to mix everything really well.

NUTRIENT-DENSE GOJI MARY

- 1 cup of coconut water
- Handful of goji berries
- ½ tsp cinnamon
- 1 Medjool date, pitted
- 1 tsp acai powder
- 2 drops food-grade lemon essential oil
- 1 tsp hemp seeds
- 1 medium stalk of celery
- Quarter of a small beetroot (or ½ tsp of beetroot powder)

Garnish with an additional small stalk of celery.

BERRY NICE

- 1 cup of coconut water
- ½ cup frozen mixed berries (organic is best)
- 6 cashews
- 1 tbsp hemp seeds
- 1 tsp maqui powder
- 1 tsp chia seeds
- 1 tsp sesame seeds
- ¼ tsp vanilla
- 2 drops food-grade wild orange essential oil

Sprinkle some cacao nibs and bee pollen on top to serve.

MEDICINAL BLUEBERRY BLITZ

- 1 cup coconut water
- ¼ cup blueberries (frozen organic)
- handful of pepitas
- 1 tsp medicinal mushroom powder
- 1 tsp organic cacao powder
- 1 tsp acai powder
- ½ tsp spirulina powder
- 2 drops food-grade copaiba essential oil
- Squirt of echinacea liquid
- Small sprig of parsley

Sprinkle cacao nibs and extra pepitas on top to serve.

IMMUNITY-BOOSTING SMOOTHIE

- 1 cup coconut water
- handful of pepitas
- handful of sunflower seeds
- ½ cup of blueberries
- 1 tsp medicinal mushroom powder
- 1 tsp camu camu powder
- 1 tsp hemp protein powder
- Sprig of parsley
- 2 drops food-grade protective blend essential oil

Sprinkle cacao nibs on top to serve.

BANANA CHOC THICKSHAKE

- 1 cup almond milk
- 1 small banana
- 1 tbsp maple syrup
- handful of sunflower seeds
- 1 Medjool date, pitted
- 1 tsp peanut butter
- 1 tsp maca powder
- 1 tsp organic cacao powder
- 1 drop food-grade cinnamon essential oil

To serve, dust some ground cinnamon on top.

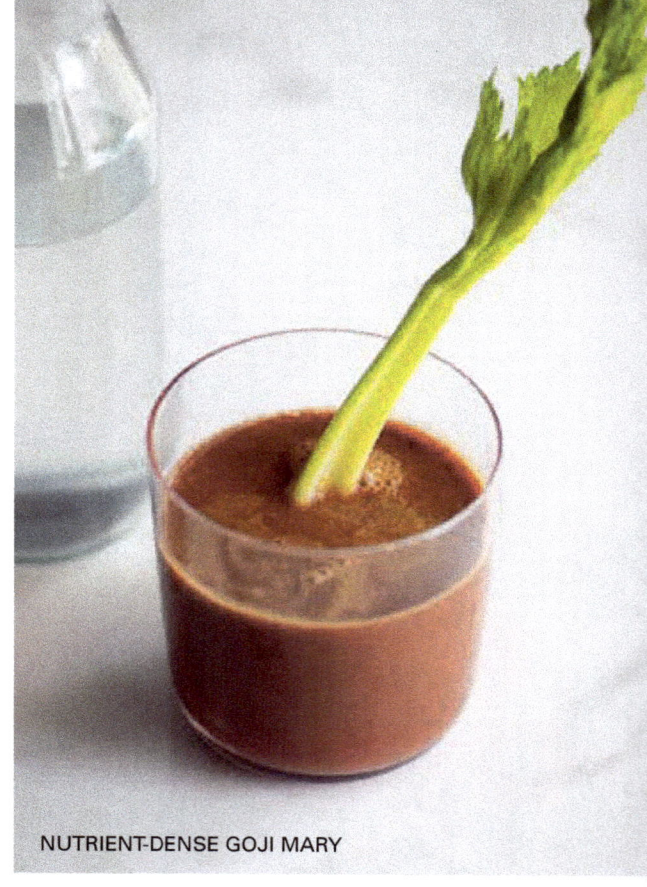

NUTRIENT-DENSE GOJI MARY

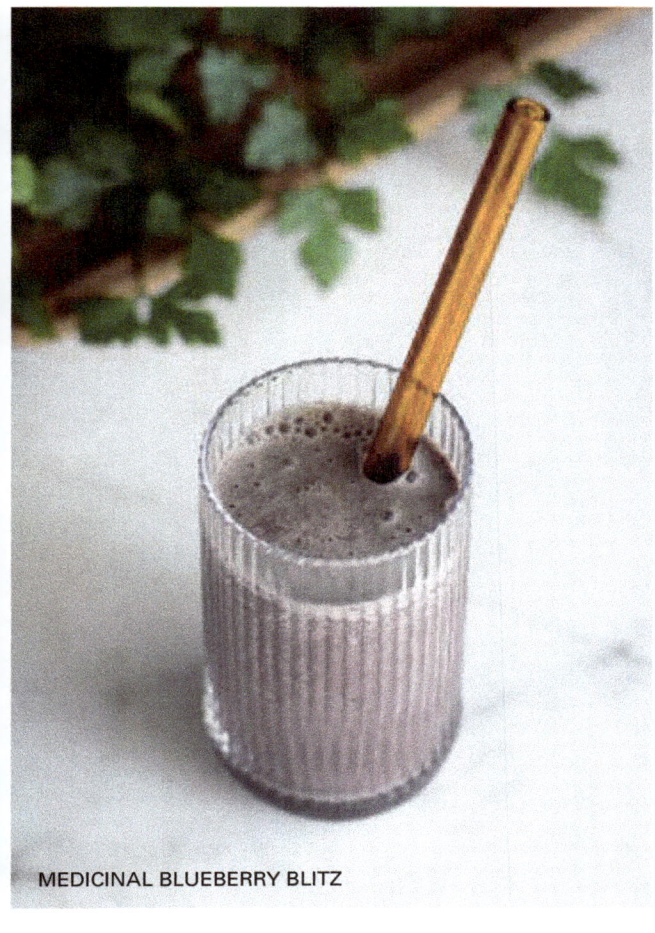

MEDICINAL BLUEBERRY BLITZ

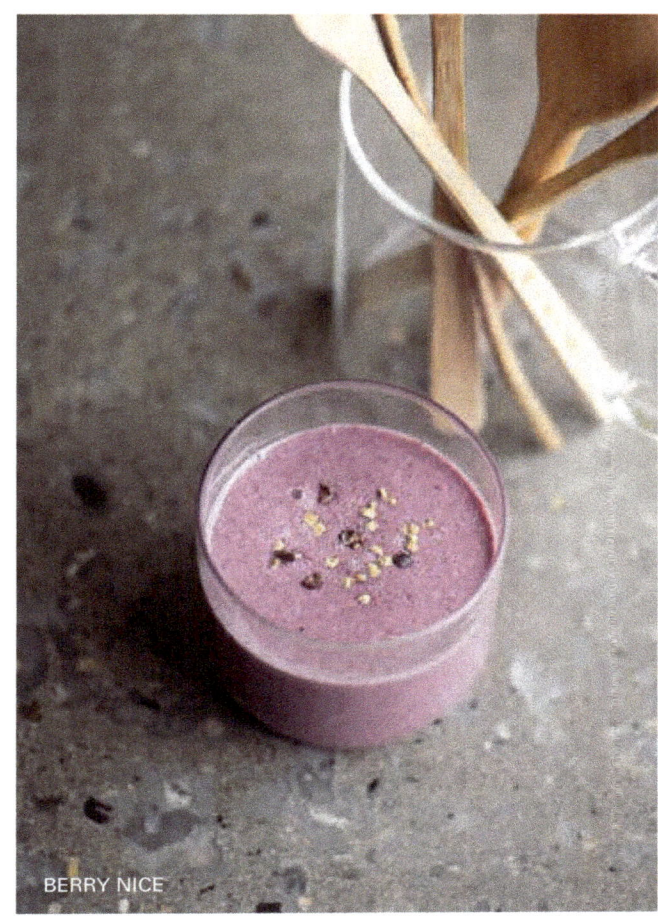

BERRY NICE

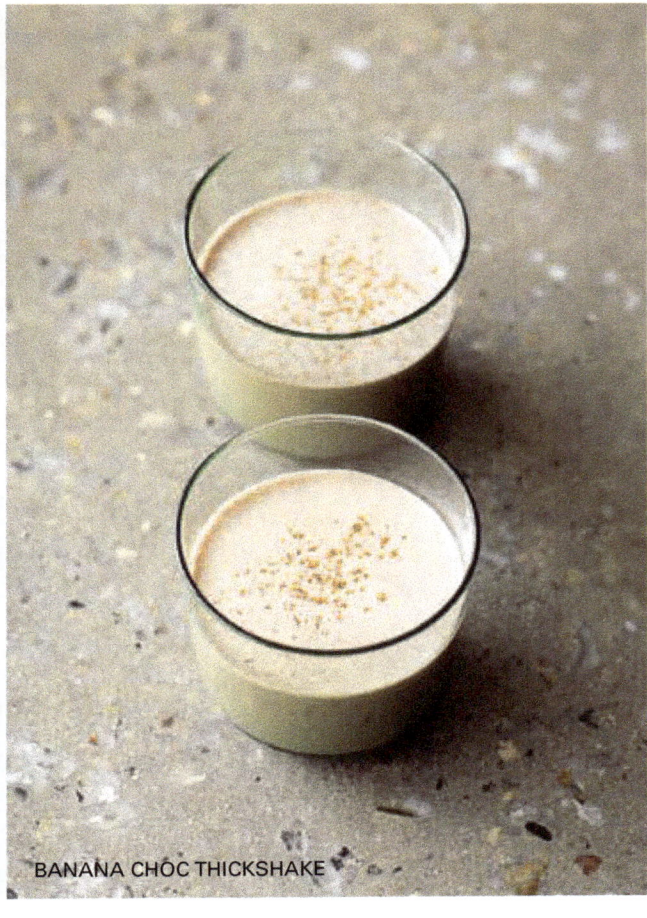

BANANA CHOC THICKSHAKE

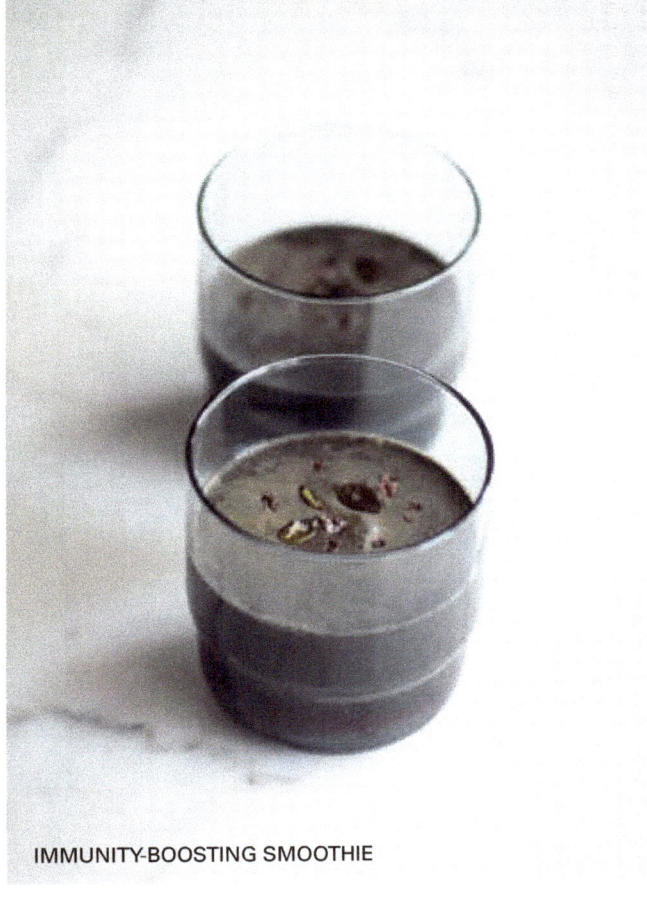

IMMUNITY-BOOSTING SMOOTHIE

THANK YOU

I firstly wish to thank my life partner and best friend Noel for believing in me. Our shared vision to make the world a better place and being able to travel and work together is just a dream come true.

To my family who have always supported and loved me in my life's choices and journey – thank you.

My cacao sister Vanessa Jean who initially introduced me to raw chocolate many years ago and inspired me to create and play with cacao, I wouldn't be writing this if it weren't for you.

To everyone in our personal and wider dōTERRA community, thank you for journeying in health with us.

To everyone who has supported us on our journey, through meditation classes, chocolate workshops and have crossed paths with us – thank you for your support and love.

To Natarsha for her epic styling, photography and concept for the book, it was dream working with you making, styling and photographing food to nostalgic tunes of our youth! And to Emma for her tireless editing and beautiful wording.

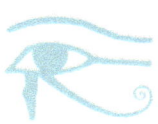

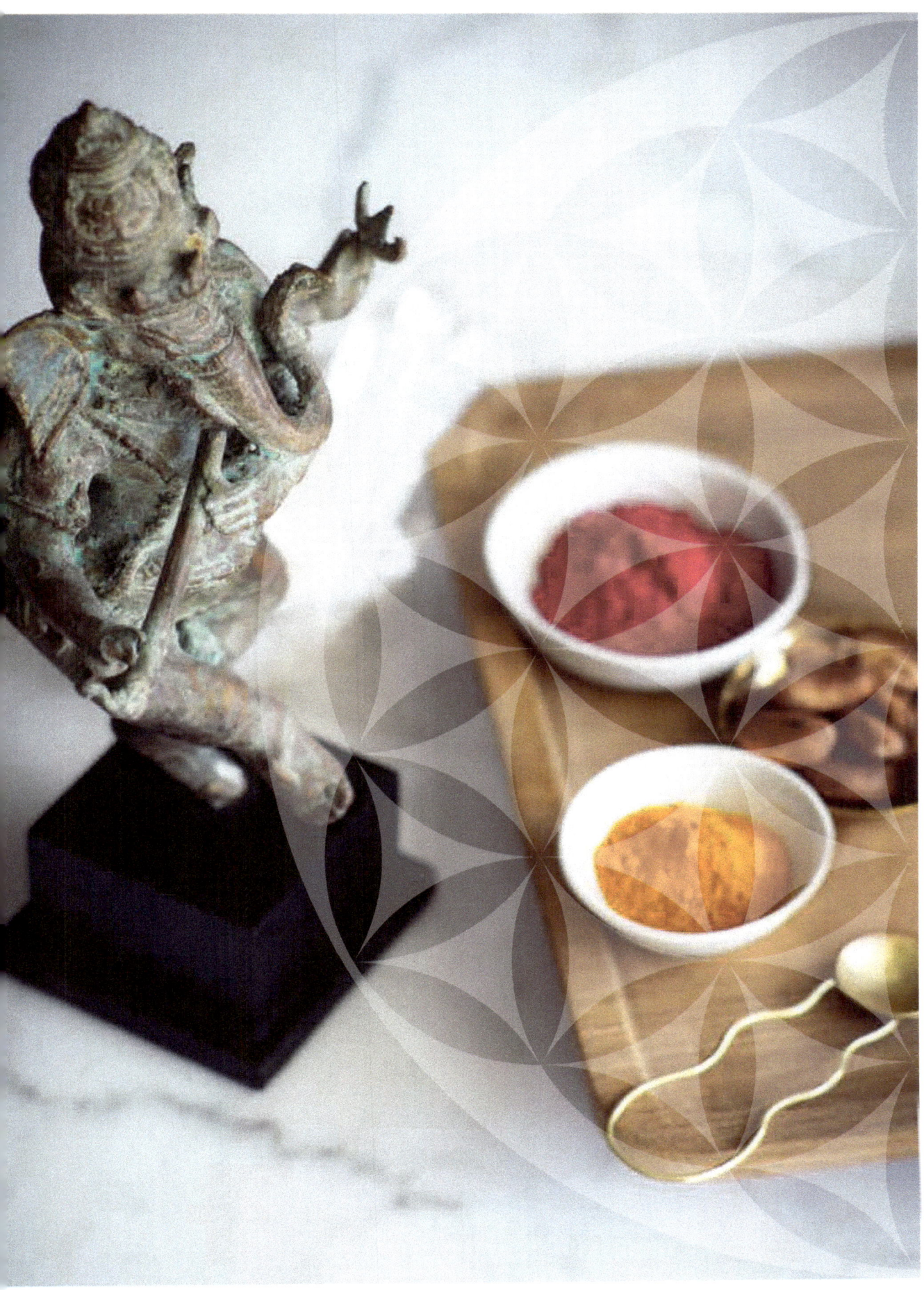

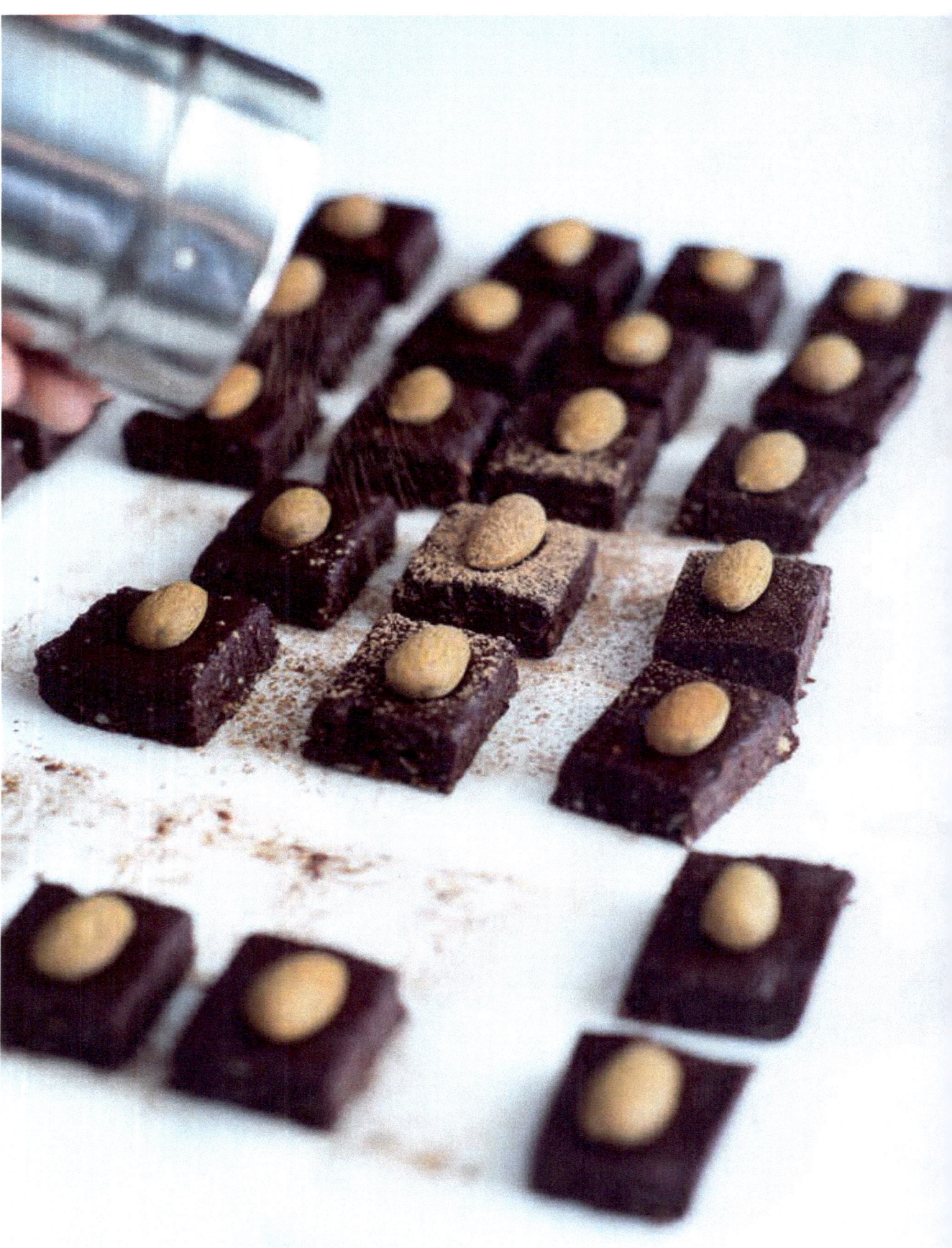

INDEX

A

Acai, about 15
   Fruit Nut Seed Clusters 104
   Macadamia Fudge with Limoncello Ganache 108
   Medicinal Blueberry Blitz 118
   Nutrient-dense Goji Mary 118
Activated Nuts, how to 25
Alcohol, in chocolates
   Espresso martini chocolates 111
   Macadamia Fudge with Limoncello Ganache 108
Almond Butter
   Cashew Lime Cups 36
   Chocolate Coated Nutty Tangerine Balls 47
   Matcha Soft Centre Chocolates 84
   Pistachio Tahini Cups 55
   Roasted Nuts in Raw Chocolate Ginger Cups 35
Almond Milk
   Banana Choc Thickshake 118
   Chia Cardamom Orange Pudding 72
Almonds
   Activated Nuts 25
   Almond Chocolate with Spiced Pistachio Crackle 60
   Black Pepper and Fennel Raw Fudge Brownie 51
   Cardamom Cacao Caramelised Roasted Nut Slab 80
   Fruit Nut Seed Clusters 104
   Hemp and Almond Ginger Lime Fudge 87
   Hemp and Matcha Cardamom Nut Balls 59
   Nuts and Seeds Chunky Pods with Coconut Cream 95
   Peppermint Hemp Balls 96
   Raw Almond Cacao Fudge 67
   Raw Chocolate Raspberry Slice 71
   Spiced Cacao Chai Balls 68
   Three Wise Men Bliss Balls 103
   Triple Layer Ginger and Lime Caramel Slice 39
Amaranth, flakes
   About 21
   Immunity Boosting Raw Cacao Cake Slab 75
   Puffed Grain Cacao Superfood Bars 56
Apricots, dried
   Fruit Nut Seed Clusters 104

B

Bananas
   Banana Choc Thickshake 118
   Raw Banana Peanut Butter Ice Cream 63
Bee Pollen, about 21
   Honey and Bee Pollen Lemon Chocolates 100
Beetroot
   Nutrient-dense Goji Mary 118
   Red Velvet Cardamom Truffles 31
Beetroot Powder
   Nuts and Seeds Chunky Pods with Coconut Cream 95
Black Pepper Essential Oil
   Black Pepper and Fennel Raw Fudge Brownie 51
   Buckini Nut Crunchy Cacao Slab 40
   Immunity Boosting Raw Cacao Cake Slab 75
   Spiced Cacao Chai Balls 68
Blueberries
   Berry nice, drink 118
   Cashew Lime Cups 36
   Immunity-boosting Smoothie 118
   Medicinal Blueberry Blitz 118
   Roasted Nuts in Raw Chocolate Ginger Cups 35

Blueberry Powder
   Nuts and Seeds Chunky Pods with Coconut Cream 95
   Peppermint Hemp Balls 96
Brazil Nuts
   Buckini Nut Crunchy Cacao Slab 40
   Cacao Butter Superfood Balls 76
Buckini
   Buckini Nut Crunchy Cacao Slab 40
   Immunity Boosting Raw Cacao Cake Slab 75
   Nuts and Seeds Chunky Pods with Coconut Cream 95
   Puffed Grain Cacao Superfood Bars 56
Buckwheat, about 21
   Buckini Nut Crunchy Cacao Slab 40
   Puffed Grain Cacao Superfood Bars 56

C

Cacao, about 11
   Basic Chocolate Recipe 28
Cacao Nibs
   Cashew Lime Cups 36
   Fruit Nut Seed Clusters 104
   Hemp and Almond Ginger Lime Fudge 87
   Macadamia Fudge with Limoncello Ganache 108
   Raw Chocolate Raspberry Slice 71
   Spiced Cacao Chai Balls 68
   Tangerine Mousse 64
Camu Camu, about 15
   Immunity Boosting Raw Cacao Cake Slab 75
   Immunity-boosting Smoothie 118
   Macadamia and Muscat Bark 43
   Puffed Grain Cacao Superfood Bars 56
Cardamom Essential Oil
   Almond Chocolate with Spiced Pistachio Crackle 60
   Cacao Elixir 116
   Cardamom Cacao Caramelised Roasted Nut Slab 80
   Chia Cardamom Orange Pudding 72
   Florentine 52
   Hemp and Matcha Cardamom Nut Balls 59
   Macadamia Fudge with Limoncello Ganache 108
   Nuts and Seeds Chunky Pods with Coconut Cream 95
   Red Velvet Cardamom Truffles 31
   Turkish Delight Minis 112
Cashews
   Berry nice, drink 118
   Cardamom Cacao Caramelised Roasted Nut Slab 80
   Cashew Lime Cups 36
   Lime and Orange Slice 44
   Matcha Soft Centre Chocolates 84
   Raw Chocolate Raspberry Slice 71
   Spiced Cashew Chia Fudge 92
Cassia Essential Oil
   Spiced Cashew Chia Fudge 92
Cayenne pepper
   Cacao Elixir 116
   Hemp Almond Ginger and Lime Fudge 87
Chia Seeds, about 19
   Berry nice, drink 118
   Cacao Butter Superfood Balls 76
   Chia Cardamom Orange Pudding 72
   Chocolate Coated Nutty Tangerine Balls 47
   Florentine 52
   Immunity Boosting Raw Cacao Cake Slab 75
   Peppermint Hemp Balls 96

INDEX

Puffed Grain Cacao Superfood Bars 56
Raw Chocolate Raspberry Slice 71
Salted Caramel Soft Centre Chocolates 115
Spiced Cacao Chai Balls 68
Spiced Cashew Chia Fudge 92
Three Wise Men Bliss Balls 103

Chocolate Moulds 25

Cinnamon Essential Oil
Almond Chocolate with Spiced Pistachio Crackle 60
Banana Choc Thickshake 118
Cacao Elixir 116
Damiana-infused Cacao Chocolates 88
Florentine 52
Fruit Nut Seed Clusters 104
Lemon Coconut Rough 107
Pistachio Tahini Cups 55
Raw Almond Cacao Fudge 67
Spiced Cashew Chia Fudge 92
Turkish Delight Minis 112

Cinnamon, ground or powder
Nutrient-dense Goji Mary 118
Nuts and Seeds Chunky Pods with Coconut Cream 95
Peppermint Hemp Balls 96
Raw Turkish Delight 99
Turkish Delight Minis 112

Coconut Cream, and paste
Cacao Elixir 116
Chia Cardamom Orange Pudding 72
Lemon Myrtle Mylk Chocolate with Inca Berries 79
Nuts and Seeds Chunky Pods with Coconut Cream 95

Coconut Milk
Nuts and Seeds Chunky Pods with Coconut Cream 95
Raw Banana Peanut Butter Ice Cream 63
Tangerine Mousse 64

Coconut, flakes
Buckini Nut Crunchy Cacao Slab 40
Cashew Lime Cups 36
Chia Cardamom Orange Pudding 72

Coconut, shredded
Buckini Nut Crunchy Cacao Slab 40
Chocolate Coated Nutty Tangerine Balls 47
Cobbers 48
Florentine 52
Fruit Nut Seed Clusters 104
Hemp and Matcha Cardamom Nut Balls 59
Immunity Boosting Raw Cacao Cake Slab 75
Lemon Coconut Rough 107
Lime and Orange Slice 44
Peppermint Hemp Balls 96
Puffed Grain Cacao Superfood Bars 56
Raw Chocolate Raspberry Slice 71
Raw Turkish Delight 99
Red Velvet Cardamom Truffles 31
Roasted Nuts in Raw Chocolate Ginger Cups 35
Salted Caramel Soft Centre Chocolates 115
Spiced Cashew Chia Fudge 92
Three Wise Men Bliss Balls 103

Coffee
Espresso martini chocolates 111

Copaiba Essential Oil
Damiana-infused Cacao Chocolates 88
Immunity Boosting Raw Cacao Cake Slab 75
Medicinal Blueberry Blitz 118

Cranberries
Cacao Butter Superfood Balls 76
Florentine 52
Raw Turkish Delight 99
Turkish Delight Minis 112

Crème de Cacao
Espresso martini chocolates 111

D, E & F

Damiana Leaves, about 21
Damiana-infused Cacao Chocolates 88

Drinks
Banana Choc Thickshake 118
Berry nice, drink 118
Cacao Elixir 116
Immunity-boosting Smoothie 118
Medicinal Blueberry Blitz 118
Nutrient-dense Goji Mary 118

Echinacea
Medicinal Blueberry Blitz 118

Essential Oils, about 12

Fennel Essential Oil
Black Pepper and Fennel Raw Fudge Brownie 51
Fennel and Sesame Chocolate
Spiced Cacao Chai Balls 68

Figs, about 19
Cacao Butter Superfood Balls 76

Frankincense Essential Oil
Three Wise Men Bliss Balls 103

Fruits, about 19

G

Ginger Essential Oil
Hemp and Almond Ginger Lime Fudge 87
Roasted Nuts in Raw Chocolate Ginger Cups 35
Spiced Cacao Chai Balls 68

Ginger, crystalised, about 21
Raw Turkish Delight 99
Turkish Delight Minis 112

Goji Berries, about 19
Cacao Butter Superfood Balls 76
Florentine 52
Nutrient-dense Goji Mary 118
Peppermint Hemp Balls 96
Raw Turkish Delight 99
Roasted Nuts in Raw Chocolate Ginger Cups 35
Turkish Delight Minis 112

H

Hazelnut Meal
Fer-RAW-Ro Cacao Bliss Balls 91

Hazelnuts
Turkish Delight Minis 112

Hemp Protein, about 15
Hemp and Matcha Cardamom Nut Balls 59
Immunity-boosting Smoothie 118

Hemp Seeds, about 19
Almond Chocolate with Spiced Pistachio Crackle 60
Berry nice, drink 118
Cacao Butter Superfood Balls 76
Chocolate Coated Nutty Tangerine Balls 47
Fer-RAW-Ro Cacao Bliss Balls 91
Fruit Nut Seed Clusters 104
Hemp and Almond Ginger Lime Fudge 87
Immunity Boosting Raw Cacao Cake Slab 75

INDEX

Nutrient-dense Goji Mary 118
Nuts and Seeds Chunky Pods with Coconut Cream 95
Peppermint Hemp Balls 96
Puffed Grain Cacao Superfood Bars 56
Spiced Cacao Chai Balls 68
Spiced Cashew Chia Fudge 92
Himalayan pink salt, about 23
Honey, about 17
    Black Pepper and Fennel Raw Fudge Brownie 51
    Cacao Butter Superfood Balls 76
    Cardamom Cacao Caramelised Roasted Nut Slab 80
    Chocolate Coated Nutty Tangerine Balls 47
    Honey and Bee Pollen Lemon Chocolates 100
    Peppermint Hemp Balls 96
    Raw Almond Cacao Fudge 67
    Roasted Nuts in Raw Chocolate Ginger Cups 35
    Tangerine Mousse 64
    Triple Layer Ginger and Lime Caramel Slice 39

I & K

Ice cream
    Raw Banana Peanut Butter Ice Cream 63
Inca Berries, about 21
    Fruit Nut Seed Clusters 104
    Lemon Myrtle Mylk Chocolate with Inca Berries 79
Kahlua
    Espresso martini chocolates 111

L

Lemon
    Lemon Coconut Rough 107
Lemon Essential Oil
    Cobbers 48
    Fer-RAW-Ro Cacao Bliss Balls 91
    Honey and Bee Pollen Lemon Chocolates 100
    Macadamia Fudge with Limoncello Ganache 108
    Matcha Soft Centre Chocolates 84
    Nutrient-dense Goji Mary 118
    Puffed Grain Cacao Superfood Bars 56
Lemon Myrtle Essential Oil
    Lemon Myrtle Mylk Chocolate with Inca Berries 79
Limoncello
    Macadamia Fudge with Limoncello Ganache 108
Lime Essential Oil
    Cashew Lime Cups 36
    Hemp and Almond Ginger Lime Fudge 87
    Lime and Orange Slice 44
    Matcha Soft Centre Chocolates 84
    Triple Layer Ginger and Lime Caramel Slice 39
LSA
    Peppermint Hemp Balls 96
Lucucma, about 15
    Cacao Butter Superfood Balls 76
    Spiced Cashew Chia Fudge 92

M, N & O

Maca, about 15
    Banana Choc Thickshake 118
    Black Pepper and Fennel Raw Fudge Brownie 51
    Cacao Elixir 116
    Damiana-infused Cacao Chocolates 88
    Fennel and Sesame Chocolate
    Fer-RAW-Ro Cacao Bliss Balls 91
    Florentine 52
    Immunity Boosting Raw Cacao Cake Slab 75
    Lime and Orange Slice 44
    Peppermint Hemp Balls 96
    Pistachio Tahini Cups 55
    Raw Almond Cacao Fudge 67
    Salted Caramel Soft Centre Chocolates 115
    Three Wise Men Bliss Balls 103
    Triple Layer Ginger and Lime Caramel Slice 39
    Turkish Delight Minis 112
Macadamia Nuts
    Cardamom Cacao Caramelised Roasted Nut Slab 80
    Macadamia and Muscat Bark 43
    Macadamia Fudge with Limoncello Ganache 108
Maple Syrup, about 17
Maqui, about 15
    Almond Chocolate with Spiced Pistachio Crackle 60
    Berry nice, drink 118
    Spiced Cacao Chai Balls 68
Matcha, about 15
    Hemp and Matcha Cardamom Nut Balls 59
    Matcha Soft Centre Chocolates 84
Medicinal Mushrooms, about 15
    Buckini Nut Crunchy Cacao Slab 40
    Damiana-infused Cacao Chocolates 88
    Immunity-boosting Smoothie 118
    Medicinal Blueberry Blitz 118
    Nuts and Seeds Chunky Pods with Coconut Cream 95
    Three Wise Men Bliss Balls 103
Medjool dates, about 19
    Banana Choc Thickshake 118
    Chocolate Coated Nutty Tangerine Balls 47
    Cobbers 48
    Fer-RAW-Ro Cacao Bliss Balls 91
    Hemp and Matcha Cardamom Nut Balls 59
    Lime and Orange Slice 44
    Macadamia Fudge with Limoncello Ganache 108
    Nutrient-dense Goji Mary 118
    Nuts and Seeds Chunky Pods with Coconut Cream 95
    Peppermint Hemp Balls 96
    Raw Chocolate Raspberry Slice 71
    Red Velvet Cardamom Truffles 31
    Salted Caramel Soft Centre Chocolates 115
    Spiced Cacao Chai Balls 68
    Three Wise Men Bliss Balls 103
    Triple Layer Ginger and Lime Caramel Slice 39
Metabolic Blend Oil
    Macadamia and Muscat Bark 43
Moulds, chocolate 25
Mousse
    Tangerine Mousse 64
Myrrh Essential Oil
    Three Wise Men Bliss Balls 103
Nuts, about 19
Orange Essential Oil
    Nuts and Seeds Chunky Pods with Coconut Cream 95

P

Parsley
    Immunity-boosting Smoothie 118
    Medicinal Blueberry Blitz 118
Pecan Nuts
    Cacao Butter Superfood Balls 76
    Cardamom Cacao Caramelised Roasted Nut Slab 80
    Fruit Nut Seed Clusters 104
    Nuts and Seeds Chunky Pods with Coconut Cream 95

INDEX

Peanut Butter
    Banana Choc Thickshake 118
    Hemp and Matcha Cardamom Nut Balls 59
    Raw Banana Peanut Butter Ice Cream 63
Pepitas
    About 19
    Cacao Butter Superfood Balls 76
    Chocolate Coated Nutty Tangerine Balls 47
    Florentine 52
    Fruit Nut Seed Clusters 104
    Hemp and Matcha Cardamom Nut Balls 59
    Immunity Boosting Raw Cacao Cake Slab 75
    Immunity-boosting Smoothie 118
    Medicinal Blueberry Blitz 118
    Roasted Nuts in Raw Chocolate Ginger Cups 35
Peppermint Essential Oil
    Buckini Nut Crunchy Cacao Slab 40
    Peppermint Hemp Balls 96
Persian Fairy Floss
    Turkish Delight Minis 112
Pistachios
    Almond Chocolate with Spiced Pistachio Crackle 60
    Cardamom Cacao Caramelised Roasted Nut Slab 80
    Pistachio Tahini Cups 55
    Raw Turkish Delight 99
    Roasted Nuts in Raw Chocolate Ginger Cups 35
    Turkish Delight Minis 112
Poppy Seeds, about 19
    Nuts and Seeds Chunky Pods with Coconut Cream 95
Protective Blend Essential Oil
    Immunity Boosting Raw Cacao Cake Slab 75
    Immunity-boosting Smoothie 118
    Spiced Cacao Chai Balls 68
Puffed Grains
    Puffed Grain Cacao Superfood Bars 56

R & S

Raspberries
    Raw Chocolate Raspberry Slice 71
Rose Essential Oil
    Pure Rose Oil Cacao 32
    Raw Turkish Delight 99
    Salted Caramel Soft Centre Chocolates 115
    Turkish Delight Minis 112
Rose Petals
    Raw Turkish Delight 99
    Turkish Delight Minis 112
Salt, pink Himalayan 23
Salted Caramel Soft Centre Chocolates 115
Sesame Seeds, about 19
    Berry nice, drink 118
    Cacao Butter Superfood Balls 76
    Chocolate Coated Nutty Tangerine Balls 47
    Fennel and Sesame Chocolate
    Fruit Nut Seed Clusters 104
    Hemp and Matcha Cardamom Nut Balls 59
    Nuts and Seeds Chunky Pods with Coconut Cream 95
Spearmint Essential Oil
    Cacao Butter Superfood Balls 76
Spirulina, about 15
    Damiana-infused Cacao Chocolates 88
    Immunity Boosting Raw Cacao Cake Slab 75
    Medicinal Blueberry Blitz 118

Sun Muscats, about 19
    Fruit Nut Seed Clusters 104
    Macadamia and Muscat Bark 43
Sunflower seeds, about 19
    Banana Choc Thickshake 118
    Cacao Butter Superfood Balls 76
    Chocolate Coated Nutty Tangerine Balls 47
    Hemp and Matcha Cardamom Nut Balls 59
    Immunity-boosting Smoothie 118
    Lemon Coconut Rough 107
    Nuts and Seeds Chunky Pods with Coconut Cream 95
    Peppermint Hemp Balls 96
    Three Wise Men Bliss Balls 103
Superfood Powders, about 15
Sweetners, about 17

T, U & V

Tahini
    About 21
    Cashew Lime Cups 36
    Matcha Soft Centre Chocolates 84
    Pistachio Tahini Cups 55
    Roasted Nuts in Raw Chocolate Ginger Cups 35
    Triple Layer Ginger and Lime Caramel Slice 39
Tangerine Essential Oil
    Chocolate Coated Nutty Tangerine Balls 47
    Tangerine Mousse 64
Turkish Delight
    Raw Turkish Delight 99
    Turkish Delight Minis 112
Turmeric, about 15
    Cacao Elixir 116
    Spiced Cashew Chia Fudge 92
    Three Wise Men Bliss Balls 103
Vanilla Vodka
    Espresso martini chocolates 111
Vanilla, about 17

W

Walnuts
    Lemon Coconut Rough 107
    Lime and Orange Slice 44
    Nuts and Seeds Chunky Pods with Coconut Cream 95
    Peppermint Hemp Balls 96
    Three Wise Men Bliss Balls 103
    Triple Layer Ginger and Lime Caramel Slice 39
White Mulberries
    About 19
    Buckini Nut Crunchy Cacao Slab 40
    Immunity Boosting Raw Cacao Cake Slab 75
Wild Orange Essential Oil
    Berry nice, drink 118
    Cacao Elixir 116
    Chia Cardamom Orange Pudding 72
    Fruit Nut Seed Clusters 104
    Hemp and Matcha Cardamom Nut Balls 59
    Lime and Orange Slice 44
    Nuts and Seeds Chunky Pods with Coconut Cream 95
    Puffed Grain Cacao Superfood Bars 56
    Raw Chocolate Raspberry Slice 71
    Raw Turkish Delight 99
    Red Velvet Cardamom Truffles 31
    Salted Caramel Soft Centre Chocolates 115
    Turkish Delight Minis 111

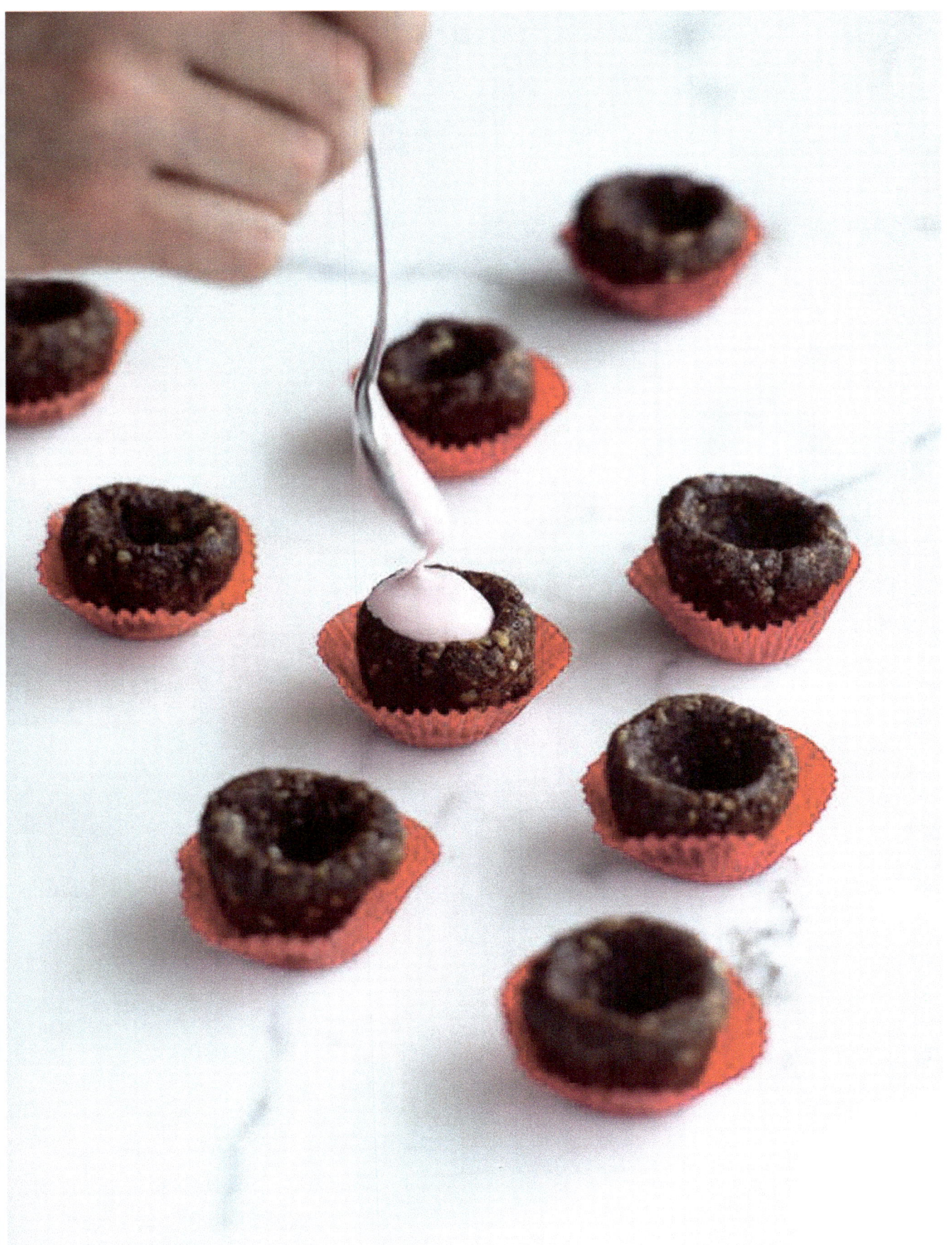

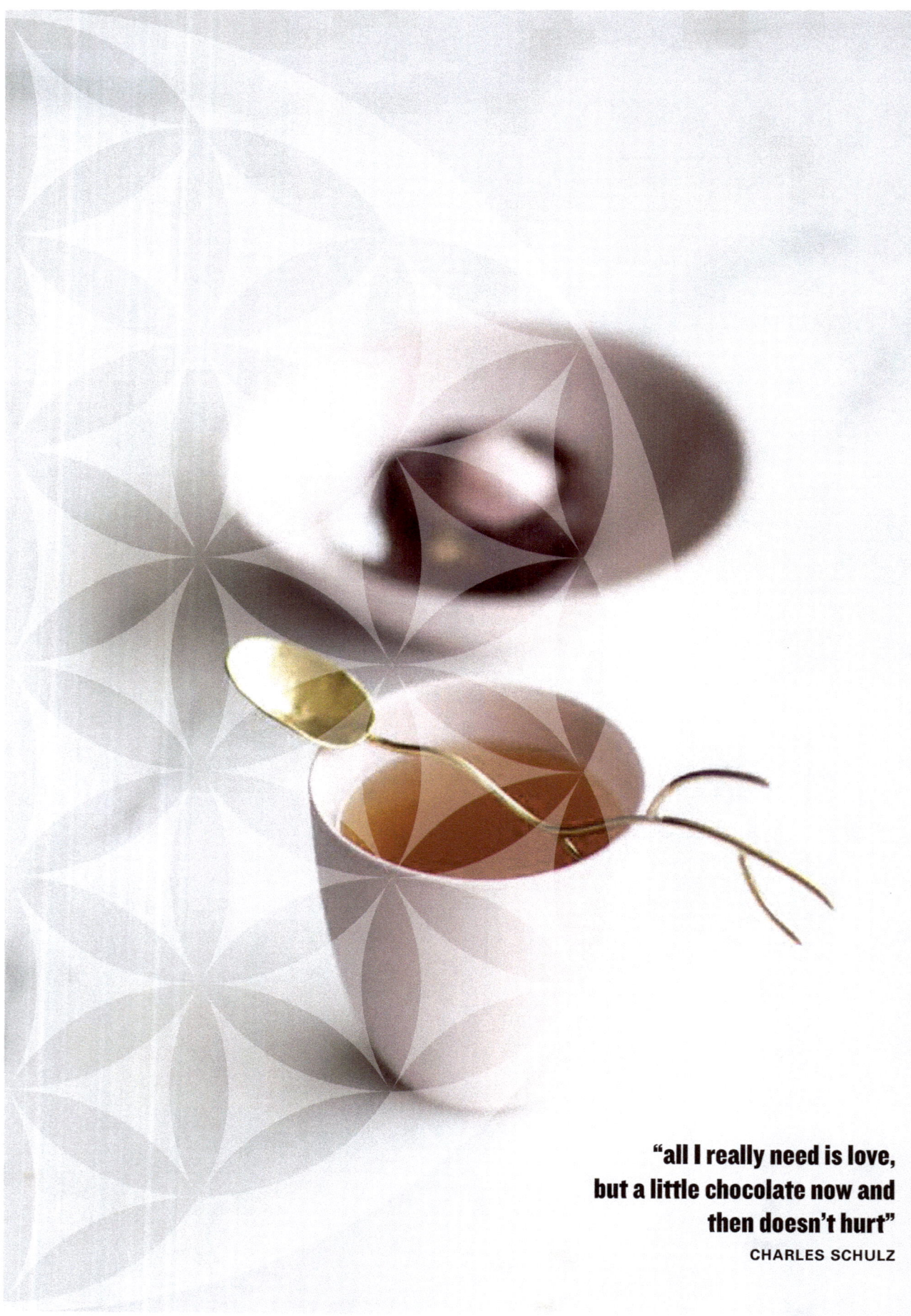

www.ingramcontent.com/pod-product-compliance
Lightning Source LLC
Chambersburg PA
CBHW061138010526
44107CB00069B/2975